W9-BBC-864

Study Guide for

Essentials for Nursing Practice

Ninth edition

Patricia A. Castaldi, DNP, RN, ANEF
Nursing Education Consultant
Winter Garden, Florida

ELSEVIER

ELSEVIER

3251 Riverport Lane
St. Louis, Missouri 63043

STUDY GUIDE FOR ESSENTIALS FOR NURSING PRACTICE, NINTH EDITION

ISBN: 978-0-323-53303-4

Copyright © 2019, Elsevier Inc. All Rights Reserved.
Previous editions copyright: 2015, 2011, 2007, 2003 by Mosby, Inc., an affiliate of Elsevier Inc.

No part of this publication may be reproduced or transmitted in any form or by any means, electronic or mechanical, including photocopying, recording, or any information storage and retrieval system, without permission in writing from the publisher. Details on how to seek permission and further information about the Publisher's permissions policies and our arrangements with organizations such as the Copyright Clearance Center and the Copyright Licensing Agency, can be found at our website: www.elsevier.com/permissions.

This book and the individual contributions contained in it are protected under copyright by the Publisher (other than as may be noted herein).

Notices

Practitioners and researchers must always rely on their own experience and knowledge in evaluating and using any information, methods, compounds or experiments described herein. Because of rapid advances in the medical sciences independent verification of diagnoses and drug dosages should be made. Fully of the law, no responsibility is assumed by Elsevier, authors, editors or contributors for any injury and/or damage to persons or property as a matter of products liability, negligence or otherwise, or from any use or operation of any methods, products, instructions, or ideas contained in the material herein.

Library of Congress Cataloging-in-Publication Data

Director: Tamara Myers
Senior Content Development Specialist: Tina Kaemmerer
Publishing Services Manager: Deepthi Unni
Project Manager: Radhika Sivalingam
Cover Design: Muthukumaran Thangaraj

Printed in the United States of America

Last digit is the print number: 9   8   7   6   5   4   3   2

Working together
to grow libraries in
developing countries

www.elsevier.com • www.bookaid.org

To John and Dan for all of your love and support. You're the best!
I couldn't do this without you!
To the faculty, students, and all of my colleagues who have inspired me throughout the years.
To all of the wonderful nurses, especially Christina and Emma, on 5 LP at
Orlando Regional Medical Center.
Thank you all for your compassion, quality care, and providing some great ideas for questions in this text!
The nurses, staff members and volunteers on 5 LP exemplify the principles of caring!

Patricia A. Castaldi

Introduction and Preface

This guide is designed to correspond, chapter by chapter, with *Essentials for Nursing Practice* (Ninth edition). Each chapter in this guide contains study aids to assist in learning and applying the theoretical concepts from the text.

The comprehensive chapter review sections allow you the opportunity to evaluate your own level of comprehension after reading the text. Use of the study group questions with fellow students may help in your overall understanding of the nursing content, as well as provide a way to further evaluate your familiarity with that content. There are also more short-answer, priority-order, and multiple-response questions to promote your preparation for classroom examinations and the alternate-format items on the NCLEX® examination. You may find that there are questions that require you to apply information from other chapters or use other reference sources to answer them. Seeking out information for patient care is a critical part of nursing practice.

General study tips to use while reading, taking classroom notes, and preparing for and taking examinations are also included in this guide. Other students have found these ideas to be helpful in their nursing course experiences.

Answers are available on the *Essentials for Nursing Practice*, ninth edition Evolve website (http://evolve.elsevier.com/Potter/essentials).

STUDY CHARTS

While reading through the chapters in the text, you may create study charts to assist you in organizing the material that is covered. The charts allow for a comparison of key concepts in the chapter. Suggestions for creating charts are provided in the chapters of this text. An example follows.

Routes of Injection

Route	Angle of Insertion/Needle Size/Maximum Amount of Medication
Intradermal	
Subcutaneous	
Intramuscular	

The learning activities presented in this study guide should assist in your review of the text material and your application of the nursing concepts to classroom and clinical experiences.

General Study Tips

When Using This Text:

- Read before the scheduled class: Highlight key points or outline content in the text that will be covered in the classroom. Don't highlight everything! Clarify with your instructor(s) what the expected readings are for your class. Tables and boxes in the text can help summarize critical information.
- Look up definitions: Find the meanings of words you do not recognize while you are going through the text. It helps to have a medical dictionary and a regular dictionary handy!
- Make notes: Write down a list of topics that you do not understand while you are reading so that you may clarify them with the instructor.
- Compare notes: Use notes taken from the book and in class to create a complete picture of the content.
- Use study/comparison charts: Put facts and ideas in an organized form so that you can refer to them easily at a later point, such as when studying for an examination.
- Use references: Go back to texts and notes used in other courses (such as anatomy and physiology) for help in understanding new material.

In the Classroom:

- Make notes: Do not try to write everything down. Note the essential information from the class. Use the margins of notebook paper or type in your mobile device any questions that you may have as you go along so that you remember to ask them at some point. Before the end of the class, note any areas that you need to clarify with the instructor.
- Ask questions: Remember to take advantage of the expertise of the instructor. Do not leave the classroom without trying to clear up areas of confusion!
- Digital recordings/Audiotape: Make recordings of classroom discussions, only with instructor permission, if:
  1. There is time to listen to them at some point (such as in the car).
  2. There are positive results from this process, with better understanding of the material and improved examination grades.

On Your Own:

- Use available resources: Take advantage of all of the resources at the school, such as the library, computer laboratory, and skill laboratory. Make time to practice nursing techniques, watch DVDs, and complete computer learning programs.

- Join/create a study group: Get together with other students in your class to review material. Study groups offer an opportunity to share information, challenge one another, and provide mutual support.
- Use time management techniques: Use available time as efficiently as possible. For example, the time that is spent waiting for an appointment or riding on public transportation may be used to read over materials or complete assignments.

Before an Exam:

- Try to remain calm: Easy to recommend but hard to do! Learn and use relaxation skills. Do not jump immediately into the examination. Relax and get focused first, then start the test.
- Be prepared: check with the instructor to be sure you have covered the content that will be on the examination. Bring the right materials: Pencils, pens, erasers, computer passwords, and so on. Leave enough time to get to the examination area so that there is no last-minute "rushing in."

During the Exam:

- Read the questions carefully: Determine what the question is asking. Stay focused on the actual question without reading into the situations. If using paper and pencil and you are allowed to mark on the examination, underline key words or cross out unnecessary information to assist in getting to the heart of the question.
- Do not keep changing your answers: Most of the time, the first answer selected is correct. Do not change an answer unless you have remembered the correct response.
- Stay focused: Take brief moments during the examination, if necessary, to stop and use relaxation techniques to compose yourself.
- For multiple response (Select All That Apply), approach each answer as being True or False in relation to the question.
- When doing the math of pharmacology, think about the answer that you obtain to see if it makes sense. How often would you give 10 tablets or 10 mL IM? If the answer does not seem realistic, recalculate!

General Suggestions for Classroom-Based and Online Courses:

- Review the syllabus in advance to identify the course requirements and expectations.

- Make a calendar to keep track of dates for examinations, quizzes, and assignments.
- Schedule time to study or complete assignments, especially if you are working.
- Connect with other students in the course electronically, by telephone, or in person.
- Take advantage of all of the available resources, such as online or on-campus tutorial programs.
- If your study habits are leading to positive results in the class, then don't make major changes. If, however, you are finding that you are not passing or just getting by in the course, you should talk with an instructor about how to change your approach in order to be more successful. Don't wait until it is too late to make a difference in your grade!
- Keep in contact with the instructor! Do not forget to ask questions.
- Maintain professional behavior with your instructors and classmates.

Contents

1   Professional Nursing

PRELIMINARY READING

Chapter 1, pp. 1–14

CASE STUDIES

1. Mr. K., a 26-year-old RN, decides that he would like to become a nurse educator.
   a. What formal education does Mr. K. need to reach this career goal?
   b. To maintain or enhance this role, what other education may be needed?

2. You are going to be interviewed for a nursing position in an extended care facility.
   a. What can you do to prepare for the interview?
   b. How can you create the best first impression?

CHAPTER REVIEW

Match the description/definition in Column A with the correct term in Column B.

	Column A	*Column B*
_____	1. Demonstrate self-care activities.	a. Communicator
_____	2. Act on behalf of the patient's interests.	b. Manager
_____	3. Provide emotional support.	c. Educator
_____	4. Coordinate members of the staff.	d. Advocate

Complete the following:

5. Identify the main purpose of the following nursing organizations:
   a. National League for Nursing (NLN)
   b. American Nurses Association (ANA)
   c. International Council of Nurses (ICN)

6. Identify four career paths that you can choose as a nurse.

7. Provide an example of how nurses and their professional organizations have lobbied at the federal or state level.

8. The three components of nursing care are:

   _____

   _____

   _____

9. Select all of the accurate statements regarding Nurse Practice Acts in the United States.

   a. Regulate the scope of practice _____

   b. Determine ethical guidelines _____

   c. Use standards from the ANA _____

   d. Vary greatly from state to state _____

   e. Originate from federal legislation _____

Copyright © 2019, Elsevier Inc. All Rights Reserved.

10. Identify four core roles for the advanced practice nurse (APRN).

11. Provide at least three examples of essential skills for nurses.

12. How can the nurse provide the patient with the best-quality care in an efficient and economically sound manner?

13. What is the difference between continuing and inservice education?

Match the description/definition in Column A with the correct person in Column B.

	Column A	Column B
_____	14. Founder of the American Red Cross.	a. Lillian Wald
_____	15. Began the Henry Street Settlement.	b. Dorothea Dix
_____	16. First professor of nursing at Columbia University.	c. Harriet Tubman
_____	17. Superintendent of the female nurses in the Union army.	d. Mary Adelaide Nutting
_____	18. Active in the Underground Railroad movement.	e. Mary Mahoney
_____	19. Founder of the Nurses' Associated Alumnae of the US and Canada.	f. Clara Barton
_____	20. First professionally educated African-American nurse.	g. Isabel Hampton Robb

21. Identify at least three external influences on the practice of nursing today.

22. Provide examples of workplace hazards that are faced by nurses.

23. Nurses recognize that the use of genomics in health care allows providers to:

24. Select all of the examples of the QSEN competency for patient-centered care:

   a. Determining the patient's meal preferences. _____

   b. Using a flowchart for the nursing care plan. _____

   c. Identifying the cultural needs of the patient. _____

   d. Documenting on the patient's electronic health record. _____

   e. Resolving a staff conflict over vacation time. _____

   f. Implementing a patient fall protocol. _____

25. How can nurses play an active role in emergency preparedness?

26. Select all of the accurate characteristics of today's health care system.

   1. Costs are decreasing. _____

   2. Over half of the US population will be part of a minority group by 2044. _____

   3. More services are hospital based. _____

   4. There are fewer underserved individuals. _____

   5. The over 65-year-old population is increasing. _____

   6. The population is shifting from urban centers to rural areas. _____

Copyright © 2019, Elsevier Inc. All Rights Reserved.

Select the best answer for each of the following questions:

27. An accurate statement regarding nursing and health care is:
    1. The majority of the public rank nurses highest among professionals for honesty.
    2. Acting in a professional manner does not have an influence on consumer perceptions of health care providers.
    3. Public policy cannot be affected by nursing involvement.
    4. There is less public access to health care information.

28. The nurse, in considering the difference between autonomy and accountability, recognizes that autonomy is:
    1. initiating nursing interventions that do not require medical orders.
    2. the legal responsibility for nursing interventions.
    3. incorporating values into practice.
    4. generating knowledge to support practice.

29. Which of the following is correct regarding the NCLEX-RN®?
    1. LPN/LVNs take the same exam.
    2. The exam includes specialty certification.
    3. It is the same requirement for all of the United States and Canada.
    4. It can be taken as many times as desired.

STUDY GROUP QUESTIONS

- How did the profession of nursing develop? Who were some of the founders of the profession?
- What are some of the major influences on nursing today?
- What is professionalism in relation to nursing? What are the characteristics of professional practice?
- How are the standards for nursing practice developed? What are the legal and ethical aspects of practice?
- What are the varied responsibilities and roles of nurses?
- How can individuals prepare to be nurses? What career opportunities are available?
- What professional nursing organizations exist and what are their goals/purposes?
- What is the role of the End-of-Life Nursing Education Consortium (ELNEC)?
- What are the current trends in nursing?
- What are the QSEN competencies and how are they incorporated into nursing practice?

STUDY CHART

Create a study chart to compare the *different levels of nursing education* and the career roles that may be attained at each level.

Copyright © 2019, Elsevier Inc. All Rights Reserved.

2 Health and Wellness

PRELIMINARY READING

Chapter 2, pp. 15–28

CASE STUDIES

1. A personal friend has been experiencing severe stomach and intestinal distress for a few months. She is 35 years old and is employed as an advertising salesperson for a local newspaper. During the past year, she has been pressured to create more income for her department. When you ask her if she has sought medical treatment, she responds, "I don't have the time to go to the doctor." In addition to her job responsibilities, she is a single parent of a grade school child who enjoys several after-school activities.
   a. What physical and lifestyle factors are present in this situation?
   b. What initial responses/interventions may be helpful for this individual?

2. Mr. G., 44 years old, has recently been diagnosed with diabetes mellitus. He requires a change in his diet and activity, and he will need to take insulin.
   a. Identify factors that could influence his coping with or managing of the disease.
   b. What illness behaviors could Mr. G. possibly demonstrate?
   c. What impact can this illness have on Mr. G.'s wife?
   d. How can the QSEN competency of safety be applied?

3. Ms. B., 55 years old, has colon cancer and is undergoing chemotherapy. Side effects of the treatment include weight loss with skin sagging, hair loss, and reduced energy. Ms. B. is an elementary school teacher with an active second-grade class.
   a. What factors are going to influence Ms. B. in coping with the illness?
   b. What are possible responses to her body image and self-concept?

CHAPTER REVIEW

Match the description/definition in Column A with the correct term in Column B.

	Column A	*Column B*
_____	1. A person's definition and interpretation of symptoms and use of the health care system	a. Health belief model
_____	2. A belief that patients have the authority to be active participants in determining their health and well-being	b. Internal variables
		c. Body image
_____	3. Longer than 6 months' duration	d. Holistic health
_____	4. A subjective concept of physical appearance	e. Illness behavior
_____	5. Developmental stage, intellectual background, emotional and spiritual factors	f. Acute illness
_____	6. Short term and severe	g. Chronic illness
_____	7. Addresses the relationship between a person's beliefs and behaviors	

Copyright © 2019, Elsevier Inc. All Rights Reserved.

Complete the following:

8. Health is the absence of disease.

   True _____ False _____

9. Identify at least one health-promotion concern for older adults.

10. Identify Maslow's hierarchy of needs on the pyramid:

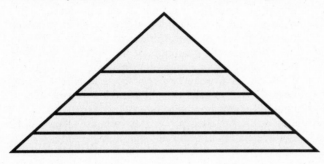

11. Identify whether the following are internal or external variables that influence health beliefs and practices.
    a. Financial status
    b. Family health behaviors
    c. Intellectual background
    d. Cultural values
    e. Developmental stage
    f. Emotions

12. Identify examples of positive and negative health behaviors.

13. Transmission of the Zika virus has been a global concern. Identify the characteristics of individuals who would most likely be motivated to follow preventive recommendations.

14. What are two goals of *Healthy People 2020*?

15. Identify all of the external variables that may influence a person's illness behaviors. Select all that apply.

    a. Visibility of symptoms _____

    b. Disruption of normal routine _____

    c. Accessibility of the health care system _____

    d. Acuity of the illness _____

    e. Cultural background _____

    f. Economics _____

16. Which of the following are risk factors that the nurse can work with the patient to modify?

    1. Genetic background _____

    2. Nutritional intake _____

    3. Excessive sun exposure _____

    4. Family medical history _____

    5. Alcohol abuse _____

Select the best answer for each of the following questions:

17. At the tertiary level of prevention, a nurse would prepare an educational program for a group requiring:
    1. chemotherapy.
    2. cardiac rehabilitation.
    3. genetic screening.
    4. sex education.

18. At the secondary level of prevention, the intervention that a nurse expects to assist with or provide instruction for is:
    1. immunization.
    2. bathing a newborn.
    3. performance of a blood test for lipid levels.
    4. referral to outpatient therapy for monitoring.

19. A nurse is working with a patient who is experiencing chronic joint pain. To assist the patient to manage or reduce the pain, the nurse decides to use a holistic health approach. With this in mind, the nurse specifically elects to include:
    1. aroma therapy.
    2. wound care.
    3. hygienic care measures.
    4. analgesic medications.

20. A nurse is completing an assessment for a patient who has gone to a medical clinic. Variables that influence the patient's health beliefs and practices are being determined. The nurse is aware that an internal variable for this patient is the:
    1. way in which the patient celebrates family occasions.
    2. manner in which the patient deals with stress on the job and at home.
    3. frequency of the family's visit to the health care agency.
    4. amount of insurance coverage that is provided by the patient's employer.

21. A nurse recognizes that primary prevention is a critical aspect in health care. The target group for a program on hand hygiene for this level of prevention is:
    1. fourth-grade children at the elementary school.
    2. patients in a cardiac rehabilitation program at the medical center.
    3. parents of a child with a congenital heart defect.
    4. patients with diabetes at the outpatient clinic.

5

Copyright © 2019, Elsevier Inc. All Rights Reserved.

22. A nurse is leading a group of community members who are trying to quit smoking. In the precontemplation phase of health behavior change, the nurse anticipates that the group members will respond by:
    1. discussing previous attempts at quitting.
    2. recognizing the benefits of not smoking.
    3. expressing irritation when the topic of quitting is introduced.
    4. requesting phone numbers of support people who have participated in the group.

23. A young adult student has gone to the university's health center for a physical examination. The nurse conducting the initial interview is looking for possible lifestyle risk factors. The nurse is specifically alerted to the student's:
    1. mild hypertension.
    2. mountain climbing hobby.
    3. family history of diabetes.
    4. part-time job at the auto factory.

24. According to Maslow's hierarchy of needs, a patient's priority should be:
    1. physical safety.
    2. psychological safety.
    3. self-esteem.
    4. adequate nutrition.

25. In preparing to teach a community group about general health promotion, the nurse recognizes that the program should focus on:
    1. providing ways for individuals to achieve control of their lives.
    2. helping people to avoid functional declines.
    3. motivating the group to reach more stable levels of wellness.
    4. giving information about specific disease processes.

26. To determine a patient's stage in the process of changing behaviors in response to being diagnosed with diabetes, a nurse can conclude that the patient is in the maintenance stage on the basis of which response?
    1. "I don't believe I need injections because I feel okay."
    2. "I may need to adjust my diet a little."
    3. "I take my insulin daily as ordered."
    4. "I have been trying to learn the diet plan."

27. A nurse recognizes an environmental risk for illness upon learning that the patient:
    1. works in a chemical plant.
    2. has a history of heart disease.
    3. admits to intermittent substance abuse.
    4. is older than 65 years of age.

STUDY GROUP QUESTIONS

- What are the different health models and how can they be applied to different patient situations? What are the advantages and disadvantages of each model?
- What are the different internal and external variables that are present in health practices and illness behavior? Give specific examples of the different variables and possible nursing interventions.
- What behaviors may be observed in a patient during illness? What impact may the patient's illness have on the family and significant others?
- How do the levels of prevention relate to the nursing care of patients in different health care settings?

STUDY CHART

Create a study chart to compare the *Levels of Prevention* that identifies both patient and nursing activities associated with each level.

Create a study chart to compare and contrast the following models: Health Beliefs, Health Promotion, Holistic Health.

Copyright © 2019, Elsevier Inc. All Rights Reserved.

3 The Health Care Delivery System

PRELIMINARY READING

Chapter 3, pp. 29–47

CASE STUDIES

1. An 80-year-old female patient has just been diagnosed with an inoperable cancerous growth in the brain. After being told of the poor prognosis, she opts to refuse chemotherapy.
   a. Where could this individual be referred for terminal care?

2. You are working on the orthopedic unit in an acute care hospital. The patient has had hip surgery and will require follow-up therapy.
   a. What kind of follow-up referral could be made?
   b. How will you use the QSEN competency of teamwork and collaboration in the management of the patient's discharge needs?
   c. What are some of the challenges that are faced in discharge planning?

CHAPTER REVIEW

Match the description/definition in Column A with the correct term in Column B.

	Column A	Column B
_____	1. Nationwide health insurance program that provides benefits to individuals older than 65 years of age	a. Medicaid
_____	2. Integration of best knowledge, clinical expertise, and patient values	b. Capitation
_____	3. Fixed amount of payment for services per enrollee	c. Globalization
_____	4. Short-term relief for persons providing care to ill, disabled	d. Magnet status
_____	5. Income eligibility for coverage below the federal poverty level	e. Parish nursing
_____	6. Reimburses health care providers for specific episodes of care, such as an inpatient hospital stay.	f. Medicare
_____	7. Nurses deliver health care services to patients within their own religious communities.	g. Respite care
_____	8. Worldwide in scope	h. Integrated delivery networks (IDNs)
_____	9. A set of providers and services organized to deliver a coordinated continuum of care to the population of patients in a specific market	i. Evidence-based
_____	10. A program to recognize health care organizations that achieve excellence in nursing practice	j. Bundled payment

Copyright © 2019, Elsevier Inc. All Rights Reserved.

Complete the following:

11. A(n) _____ is a system of family-centered care designed to allow patients to live with dignity while dealing with a terminal illness.

12. a. What are the key elements in discharge planning?

    b. When should discharge planning begin in the acute care setting?

13. Identify examples of technological advances that influence health care delivery.

14. What are the eight principles of patient-centered care?

15. Select the appropriate health care service level for each of the following (selections may be used more than once):

    Well-baby care _____

    Intensive care treatment _____

    Cardiac rehabilitation program _____

    Visiting nurses _____

    Adult day care center _____

    Immunizations _____

    Family planning clinic _____

    Mental health counseling _____

    Appendectomy surgery _____

    Assisted-living facility _____

    CT scans _____

    Sports medicine _____

    a. Primary care
    b. Secondary acute care
    c. Preventive care
    d. Tertiary care
    e. Restorative care
    f. Continuing care

16. A role of a case manager is to:

17. The average length of stay (LOS) in an acute care hospital is: _____

18. Based on the dimensions of patient-centered care, select all of the following that patients want specifically with regard to *access* to health care.
    a. To schedule appointments at convenient times without difficulty _____
    b. To have a setting that focuses on the quality of life _____
    c. To receive accurate and timely information _____
    d. To have an environment that is clean and comfortable _____
    e. To see a specialist when a referral is made _____
    f. To interact with a competent and caring staff _____
    g. To find transportation when going to different health care settings _____
    h. To have family members involved in the plan of care _____

19. What is involved in the process of patient referrals?

20. The Patient Protection and Affordable Care Act of 2010 focuses on:

21. Identify four areas that are part of the Minimum Data Set for Resident Assessment.

22. One of the biggest drawbacks of assisted living facilities is: _____

23. Health care reform stimulated the development of these two systems:

    _____

    _____

Copyright © 2019, Elsevier Inc. All Rights Reserved.

24. What services does a nursing center provide? Select all that apply.

    a. 24-hour intermediate care _____

    b. Dietary management _____

    c. Acute care services _____

    d. An interdisciplinary approach _____

    e. Focus on a young adult patient population _____

25. Identify two ways that health care agencies demonstrate quality and safety:

    _____

    _____

26. Identify the characteristics of a critical access hospital: Select all that apply.
    a. It provides services during daytime hours only.

    _____

    b. Basic laboratory services are offered. _____

    c. There are usually more than 200 beds. _____

    d. Temporary care is provided for 96 hours or less.

    _____

    e. Staffing consists primarily of RNs and CNAs

    _____

27. Identify how patient satisfaction is linked to health care finances.

28. What are some of the factors contributing to the predicted expansion of the nursing shortage?

29. What is OASIS and what are three (3) of the data items within it?

30. What is the Hospital Consumer Assessment of Healthcare Providers and Systems (HCAHPS)?

Select the best answer for each of the following questions:

31. The daughter of an older woman expresses her concern that while the daughter is at work her mother, recently diagnosed with Alzheimer's disease, has been found wandering around the neighborhood in a disoriented state. This family may benefit from the services of a(n):
    1. hospice.
    2. subacute care unit.
    3. adult day care center.
    4. residential community.

32. While working in the community health agency, a nurse visits an older adult patient who is having difficulty performing activities of daily living (ADLs) in her own home. The patient recognizes that she needs some supervision with medications. In discussions with this patient, the nurse refers the patient to a(n):
    1. subacute care unit.
    2. assisted-living facility.
    3. rehabilitation hospital.
    4. primary care institution.

33. A patient is discharged from a medical unit and requires more constant nursing care at a level above a nursing center or extended care facility. The nurse recognizes that this patient will be referred to a(n):
    1. subacute care unit.
    2. home health care agency.
    3. urgent care center.
    4. rural primary care facility.

34. A nurse's next-door neighbor has recently experienced some health problems. The neighbor visits the nurse to ask about Medicaid coverage. The nurse informs the neighbor that this program is:
    1. catastrophic long-term care coverage for older adults.
    2. a fee-for-service plan that provides preventive health care.
    3. a two-part federally funded health care program for older adults.
    4. a federally funded and state-regulated program for individuals of all ages with low income.

35. A graduate of a nursing program is interested in the occupational health field. The graduate nurse decides to pursue a position at:
    1. the local medical center.
    2. a car manufacturing plant.
    3. an urgent care center.
    4. a physician's office.

9

Copyright © 2019, Elsevier Inc. All Rights Reserved.

36. A patient is being discharged from the medical unit of the hospital. While working with the patient, the nurse identifies that intermittent supervision will be required. The patient will also need to rent durable medical equipment for use in the home. There is family support for the patient upon discharge. The nurse will refer this patient to a(n):
    1. subacute care unit.
    2. extended care facility.
    3. home health agency.
    4. urgent care center.

37. The family of a patient has requested that the hospice agency become involved with the patient's care. The nurse recognizes that the services provided by hospice for this patient include:
    1. extensive rehabilitative measures.
    2. daytime coverage for the working caregivers.
    3. residential care with an emphasis on a return to functioning.
    4. provision of symptom management and comfort measures for the terminally ill.

38. Health care costs are generally less when a patient is able to be treated in a(n):
    1. outpatient setting.
    2. acute care facility.
    3. assisted living facility.
    4. specialized hospital setting.

39. When an individual is required to reimburse the health care provider for each aspect of care performed. this is termed:
    1. managed care.
    2. preferred provider.
    3. pay-for-coordination.
    4. fee-for-service.

STUDY GROUP QUESTIONS

- What types of health care financing are available, who is eligible, and what services are covered?
- What does managed care mean to patients and health care providers?
- According to the health care services levels, what health care agencies and services are available, and what are the usual roles for nurses in each agency?
- What are some of the key competencies required of nurses today?
- What processes are in place to measure health care agency quality, services, and patient satisfaction?

STUDY CHART

Create a study chart to compare the *Types of Health Care Delivery Agencies* that identifies the different health care services provided and the nursing roles and activities for each.

Copyright © 2019, Elsevier Inc. All Rights Reserved.

4 Community-Based Nursing Practice

PRELIMINARY READING

Chapter 4, pp. 48–58

CASE STUDIES

1. A nurse lives in a community that has had a steady increase in the number of older adult residents. The nurse has been approached by some of these residents and asked a variety of health-related questions. The nurse decides to investigate the needs of older adults and the resources available to this population.
   a. For the older adult, what problems and needs should the nurse anticipate?
   b. What kind of programs or services may be available or could be offered in this community for the older adult residents?

2. A 54-year-old patient was discharged from the medical center after being diagnosed with diabetes mellitus. The patient will be taking oral medication and needs to maintain dietary restrictions. Patient teaching was started during the brief stay in the medical center, but the discharge planning nurse has contacted the community health agency to follow up with the patient. You will be visiting this patient in his home today.
   a. What should you include in the assessment of the patient's home environment?
   b. What assessment data will you need to obtain from the patient?

3. There are a number of homeless residents who come to the community health clinic.
   a. What specific considerations are required for a homeless patient who has a chronic illness?

CHAPTER REVIEW

Complete the following:

1. The focus of community-based care is to:

2. One challenge for community-based health care is:

3. The difference between public health and community health nursing is:

4. Identify a particular risk for individuals from the following vulnerable populations:
   a. Immigrant
   b. Poor and homeless
   c. Mentally ill
   d. Older adult

5. Identify the role of the nurse in community-based practice for each of the following examples:
   a. Coordinating the visits of physical and occupational therapists _____

   b. Demonstrating the use of an aerosol nebulizer _____

   c. Collecting and analyzing data to identify disease trends _____

6. What are the three components or parts of a community?

   _____

   _____

   _____

7. Identify three interventions for a family with a member who is dealing with substance abuse.

Copyright © 2019, Elsevier Inc. All Rights Reserved.

8. Specify four interventions for a patient with Alzheimer's disease.

9. Identify potential safety hazards in the photo below:

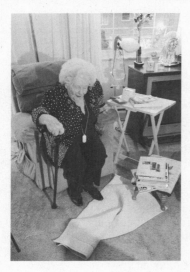

10. Provide examples of incidence rates in the community that could be researched by the nurse.

11. Specific health care risks for the immigrant population include (select all that apply):

   a. Diabetes mellitus _____

   b. Tuberculosis _____

   c. Heart disease _____

   d. Hepatitis B _____

   e. Dental problems _____

   f. Urinary infection _____

12. What data can be collected when the nurse performs a "windshield survey"?

Select the best answer for each of the following questions:

13. A nurse is aware that the homeless population has a higher prevalence of:
   1. diabetes mellitus.
   2. heart disease.
   3. mental illness.
   4. asthma.

14. A nurse is working with a member of a vulnerable population within the community. Which intervention should be completed first?
   1. Providing financial advice
   2. Setting all of the priorities for the patient and family
   3. Performing a long and detailed family assessment
   4. Considering the meaning of the patient's language and behavior

15. In completing an assessment of a community's social system, the nurse investigates the
   1. schools.
   2. economy.
   3. educational level of the population.
   4. distribution of the population by age.

16. For an older adult with a cognitive impairment living in the community, a nurse should specifically plan to
   1. provide a well-lighted, glare-free environment.
   2. promote activities that reinforce reality.
   3. make arrangements for a hearing evaluation.
   4. encourage the use of self-help groups.

STUDY GROUP QUESTIONS

- What are the essential functions of public and community health?
- How does the community health nurse care for the community?
- What competencies are required of a community health nurse?
- What roles are assumed by the community health nurse?
- What are the special needs of vulnerable populations?
- How does the nurse approach and care for vulnerable populations?
- What is included in the assessment of the community?

Copyright © 2019, Elsevier Inc. All Rights Reserved.

5 Legal Principles in Nursing

PRELIMINARY READING

Chapter 5, pp. 59–72

CASE STUDIES

1. In preparation for surgery, you are to have the patient sign the consent form for the procedure. During discussions about postoperative care, the patient does not appear to fully understand what will be done during the surgery.
   a. What are your responsibilities in this situation?

2. You are reviewing the doctor's orders for the medications to be given to the patient. One of the medication orders is very difficult to read. The nurse in charge tells you that she is sure it is Lasix 40 mg PO.
   a. What should you do in this circumstance?
   b. What legal implications may be involved if the order is incorrect?

3. A child arrives in the emergency department in critical condition. His parents are divorced.
   a. What issues concerning consent for treatment may be involved in this child's case?

4. You have been observing a nursing colleague on your unit, and she appears to be taking narcotics from the medication cart. There have been occasions when her behavior has been erratic.
   a. What, if any, are your legal responsibilities regarding this colleague's behavior?

5. You are looking at a popular social media site and notice that a staff member has posted photos of a patient without permission.
   a. What should you do?
   b. What are the possible consequences of the nurse's action?

CHAPTER REVIEW

Match the descriptions/definitions in Column A with the correct term in Column B.

Column A	Column B
_____ 1. Completed when anything unusual happens that could potentially cause harm to a patient, visitor, or employee	a. Tort
_____ 2. Any willful attempt or threat to harm another person	b. Negligence
_____ 3. A civil wrong or injury for which remedy is in the form of money damages	c. Living wills
_____ 4. A crime of a serious nature that usually carries a penalty of imprisonment	d. Statutory law
_____ 5. Limitation of liability for health care professionals offering assistance at the scene of an accident	e. Good Samaritan law
_____ 6. Conduct that falls below the standard of care	f. Assault
_____ 7. Any intentional touching of another person's body without consent	g. Common law
_____ 8. A form of contemporary laws created by elected legislative bodies	h. Battery
_____ 9. Documents instructing physicians to withhold or withdraw life-sustaining procedures	i. Incident or occurrence report
_____ 10. A form of contemporary law created by judicial decision in court when cases are decided	j. Felony

13

Copyright © 2019, Elsevier Inc. All Rights Reserved.

Complete the following:

11. The best way for a nurse to avoid being liable for negligence is to:

12. Identify two areas in which standards of care are defined.

13. a. Informed consent requires that the patient:

    b. For informed consent, the nurse's role is to:

14. A 9-year-old boy arrives at the hospital after a fall from a tree. He will need emergency surgery. The 25-year-old brother who has brought him to the hospital may give legal consent.

    True _____ False _____

15. Identify where information on the Nursing Licensure Compact (NLC) may be found.

16. Select from the following all of the correct statements regarding the Good Samaritan Law (1998):
    a. Health care providers are not liable for care provided during an emergency, even if they are not trained in the care they offer. _____
    b. In an emergency, nurses may treat minors without a parent's consent. _____
    c. Health care providers must follow through on care that is provided in an emergency, transferring the victim to EMTs or other emergency personnel. _____

17. A verbal or telephone order from a physician usually needs to be signed within _____ hours.

18. The two standards for determination of death are:

19. For the following, indicate if the nurse's license may be in jeopardy.
    a. The nurse is found to be driving under the influence.
    b. The nurse receives a misdemeanor traffic violation for speeding.

20. The elements of negligence/malpractice are:
    a. _____
    b. _____
    c. _____
    d. _____

21. The coroner is notified if the patient's death is:

    _____

22. Which of the following constitute a felony related to the Nurse Practice Act (select all that apply):
    a. Giving the wrong medication to a patient. _____
    b. Practicing without a license. _____
    c. Misusing controlled substances. _____
    d. Not instituting safety protocols. _____
    e. Sharing the patient's information with a co-worker. _____

23. Advance directives act to:

24. Health care workers are required to report what occurrences/incidents?

25. The parents have refused medically necessary treatment for their child. What, if anything, may be done in this circumstance?

26. A statute that encourages a health care provider to disclose patient care errors without admitting liability is called a(n): _____.

27. Malpractice insurance carriers are required by law to report insurance settlements and verdicts to the: _____.

Copyright © 2019, Elsevier Inc. All Rights Reserved.

28. Which of the following are examples of "never events" or preventable errors? Select all that apply.

    a. Patient falls. _____

    b. Urinary tract infections. _____

    c. Lost patient articles. _____

    d. Omission of a drug dosage. _____

    e. Intermittent catheterizations. _____

    f. Pressure ulcers. _____

29. Regulations specify that the use of physical or chemical restraint requires: _____.

30. The Patient Self-Determination Act (1991) requires that health care institutions:

31. Identify at least three common sources of negligence.

32. The Health Insurance Portability and Accountability Act of 1996 (HIPAA) sets standards for:

33. Indicate a circumstance on a medical center patient unit where a rapid improvement event or assessment may be used to improve care.

34. Information on continuing education requirements for initial and ongoing nursing licensure can be found at/on:

Select the best answer for each of the following questions:

35. A clinical experience is planned for an acute care facility. The student nurse recognizes that his or her liability for patient care includes:
1. no individual responsibility for actions while being supervised.
2. a shared responsibility with instructor, staff member(s), and health care agency.
3. activities performed while working in another capacity, such as a nursing assistant.
4. accountability for information and techniques that will be learned in the school.

36. There has been a serious flu epidemic among the staff at a medical center. Upon arriving to work on the medical unit, a nurse discovers that all other nursing staff members have called in sick and there are no other nurses available in the facility. In this situation, the nurse should:
1. not accept the assignment and leave the unit.
2. accept the assignment and identify the poor staffing in each patient's record.
3. document the situation and provide a copy to nursing administration.
4. inform the hospital administration that nursing responsibilities have been delegated to other personnel.

37. While a nurse is preparing to administer medication, the patient states that he or she refuses the medication. The nurse knows that the medication is important for the patient and proceeds with the injection of the medication. This is considered:
1. invasion of privacy.
2. negligence.
3. assault.
4. battery.

38. The urgent care center in town is busy this evening. There are many walk-in patients of different ages waiting for treatment. The nurse recognizes that in a nonemergency situation the individual who may give consent for a treatment is:
1. a teenage parent.
2. the grandparent of a minor.
3. a 16-year-old student.
4. the 14-year-old brother of a patient.

39. A nurse observes the following actions and recognizes that a violation of HIPAA has occurred when another nurse:
1. shares patient data with other agency personnel not involved in the patient's treatment.
2. withholds the patient's diagnosis from the family members per the patient's request.
3. provides details of a major scientific advancement to the public relations department.
4. reports an incidence of an infectious disease to the health department.

40. A nurse enters the room of a patient and observes that the patient is on the floor and an incident has occurred. The situation is appropriately documented as follows:
1. "Patient fell out of bed. Physician notified."
2. "Patient found on floor. Laceration to forehead."
3. "Patient given incorrect medication, became dizzy, and slid to the floor."
4. "Patient got out of bed without assistance and appears to have fallen."

15

Copyright © 2019, Elsevier Inc. All Rights Reserved.

41. While working as a receptionist in a physician's office, a student nurse is offered the opportunity to provide an injection to one of the patients. This individual's liability is based upon the:
   1. job description of a receptionist.
   2. educational level achieved in the nursing program.
   3. physician's willingness to accept responsibility for this individual.
   4. limits of the malpractice insurance held by the physician and this individual.

42. A nurse has administered a medication to a patient with a documented allergy to that medication. A standard of care is applied when:
   1. there is a determination of an injury to the patient.
   2. an amount of financial compensation is determined.
   3. criminal statutes from the federal government are investigated.
   4. the nurse's action is compared to that of another nurse in a similar circumstance.

43. Of the following actions, which one is considered to be assault?
   1. A nurse threatens to administer medication to a patient who refuses it.
   2. A surgeon operates on the wrong leg.
   3. A nurse fails to use aseptic technique.
   4. A nursing assistant restrains a confused patient.

44. The National Organ Transplant Act (1984) allows for or requires:
   1. physicians who certify death to participate in organ removal and transplant.
   2. health care agency removal of organs with the family's consent.
   3. donor transplant without the patient's consent.
   4. immunity from liability for the donor's estate.

45. The patient comes into the medical center with an inflammation on the right wrist. The nurse has been taking vital signs and notes that the fingers on the patient's right hand are becoming swollen and darker in color, and the patient identifies feeling "numb." The nurse has attempted to contact the prescriber two times within the last half hour without success. The nurse's first action should be to:
   1. contact the nursing supervisor to request assistance in getting medical intervention.
   2. continue to record vital signs and observations.
   3. try again to contact the patient's prescriber.
   4. document information in the patient's record.

STUDY GROUP QUESTIONS

- What are the sources and types of laws?
- What are intentional and unintentional torts?
- How may intentional torts be applied to nursing situations?
- What criteria are necessary for negligence/malpractice to occur?
- How are the standards of care defined and applied?
- Which individuals may give consent for treatment?
- What is the role of a nurse in obtaining consent?
- What is the role of a nurse in situations related to death and dying, employment contracts, and organ and tissue donation?
- How can a nurse minimize his/her liability?
- What situations require reporting by a nurse?
- How is the profession and practice of nursing influenced by legal issues?
- What are some of the legal concerns for nurses working in specialty areas, such as obstetrics?

STUDY CHART

Create a study chart describing *How to Minimize Liability* that identifies the nursing actions that reduce possible liability for the following situations: short staffing, floating, patient occurrences, and reporting/recording.

Copyright © 2019, Elsevier Inc. All Rights Reserved.

6 Ethics

PRELIMINARY READING

Chapter 6, pp. 73–82

CASE STUDIES

1. You are the home care nurse for a 42-year-old male patient who has severe multiple sclerosis. He tells you on several occasions that he is tired of living this way, of not being able to do anything for himself. He says that he has read about individuals who have been "helped to die," and he asks if you can assist him in finding out more about this procedure.
   a. Apply the steps for processing an ethical dilemma to this situation.
   b. What is the role of the nurse in this situation?

2. The son of one of your patients asks you if he can look at his mother's medical record. He insists that he needs to know what is happening so that he and his sister can plan for their mother's care.
   a. What should you do in this circumstance?

CHAPTER REVIEW

Match the description/definition in Column A with the correct term in Column B.

	Column A	Column B
_____	1. Supporting the patient's right to decision making	a. Ethics
_____	2. Considering the patient's best interest	b. Fidelity
_____	3. Avoiding deliberate harm	c. Justice
_____	4. Keeping promises	d. Morals
_____	5. Determining the order in which patients should be treated	e. Bioethics
_____	6. Consideration of standards of conduct	f. Autonomy
_____	7. Ethics within the field of health care	g. Beneficence
_____	8. Judgment about behavior	h. Nonmaleficence
_____	9. Personal beliefs about the worth of an idea, custom, or object	i. Values

Complete the following:

10. How can access to the patient's medical record become an ethical issue?

11. Identify an end-of-life issue that has ethical implications for nurses.

12. Identify the ethical theory for each of the following descriptions:
    a. This approach to ethical discourse depends on finding consensus more than an appeal to philosophic principles.
    b. Proposes that actions are right or wrong based on the essence of right and wrong in the principles of fidelity, truthfulness, and justice
    c. Discusses how ethical decisions affect women
    d. Proposes that the value of something is based on its usefulness
    e. Guides us to examine motives even as we try to establish principles of right action

Copyright © 2019, Elsevier Inc. All Rights Reserved.

13. For the following areas, provide a specific example of how ethical concerns may be involved:
    a. Cost containment
    b. Cultural sensitivity

14. In applying the QSEN competency of informatics, explain how the digital transmission of patient information can be an ethical concern.

15. Briefly describe the Capabilities Approach and how disability is seen within an ethical perspective.

Select the best answer for each of the following questions:

16. A professional code of ethics includes:
    1. legal standards for practice.
    2. extensive details on moral principles.
    3. guidelines for approaching common ethical dilemmas.
    4. a collective statement of group expectations for behavior.

17. By administering necessary medication to a patient on a unit in an extended care facility, a nurse is applying the ethical principle of:
    1. justice.
    2. fidelity.
    3. autonomy.
    4. beneficence.

18. A nurse has been working with a patient who had abdominal surgery. The patient is experiencing discomfort and has been calling often for assistance. The ethical principle of fidelity is demonstrated when the nurse:
    1. changes the dressing.
    2. provides a warm lotion back rub.
    3. informs the patient of the actions of the medications administered.
    4. returns to assist the patient with breathing exercises at the agreed-upon times.

19. A student nurse is assigned to work with parents who refuse to have essential medical treatment provided to their child. The medical center is pursuing a court order to force the family to accept the treatment plan that will assist the child. The nurse has strong feelings for the family's position, as well as the importance of the medical treatment. The first step for the nurse to take in attempting to resolve this ethical dilemma is to:
    1. examine personal values.
    2. evaluate the outcomes.
    3. gather all of the facts.
    4. verbalize the problem.

20. An example of advocacy in nursing practice is:
    1. documenting care provided to a patient.
    2. giving medication to a patient.
    3. assessing the patient's comfort level after surgery.
    4. contacting the physician to discuss the patient's response to the plan of care.

21. The last phase in the processing of an ethical dilemma is to:
    1. evaluate the action taken.
    2. consider treatment options.
    3. negotiate the options and outcomes.
    4. identify the problem.

22. Which one of the following situations represents an ethical rather than a legal consideration?
    1. Administering medications.
    2. Providing care to someone without health insurance.
    3. Sharing patient information with another health care worker.
    4. Reporting a communicable disease to the public health officer.

23. The patient asks for you to be a "friend" on Facebook. Your best response is to:
    1. say "yes" but keep your conversations private.
    2. tell him that you don't use that social media site.
    3. say "no" because it is not legal for nurses to do.
    4. thank him for the offer, but explain that you have a professional responsibility to be fair to all of your patients, as well as meet professional standards.

24. Underlying the principles of ethics is the nurse's role as a(n):
    1. advocate.
    2. educator.
    3. manager.
    4. counselor.

STUDY GROUP QUESTIONS

- What are ethics and what is the purpose of a code of ethics in a profession?
- What principles are promoted in a profession?
- How can a nurse be a patient advocate?
- What are the basic standards of ethics?
- What are values and how are they developed?
- How do values relate to ethics?
- How does a professional determine that an ethical dilemma exists?
- What are the steps for processing an ethical dilemma?
- What ethical dilemmas may arise in health care and nursing practice?

STUDY CHART

Create a study chart to identify and compare *Responsibility, Accountability, Confidentiality, Competence, Judgment, and Advocacy* and provide examples of nursing behaviors for each.

Copyright © 2019, Elsevier Inc. All Rights Reserved.

7 Evidence-Based Practice

PRELIMINARY READING

PRELIMINARY READING

Chapter 7, pp. 83–99

CASE STUDIES

1. You are working in a home care agency. One of your assigned patients is having difficulty with managing his daily insulin intake. You discover that he is having difficulty in getting an accurate blood glucose reading with his monitor. Because of the problem, the patient is self-administering too much or too little insulin. You remember that some of the other home care patients are also having some trouble with this particular glucose monitor.
   a. Use the PICO format to develop a possible question.
   b. What type of trigger is present in this scenario?

2. As a nurse for a surgical unit in a local medical center, you will be involved in identifying some quality improvement (QI) projects for your unit.
   a. What possible areas may be important for you, your fellow staff members, and the patients on your unit?

3. The nurses on the outpatient oncology infusion unit recognize that hand hygiene is critical to preventing the spread of infection. It is decided that this will be a critical focus for all of the staff and 100% compliance is expected.
   a. What type of trigger is present in this scenario?
   b. What type of data would be collected?

CHAPTER REVIEW

Match the description/definition in Column A with the correct term in Column B.

	Column A	Column B
_____	1. Characteristics or traits that vary among subjects	a. Pilot
_____	2. Prediction made about the relationship between study variables	b. Abstract
_____	3. To trial a new practice	c. Literature review
_____	4. Brief summary of an article that quickly tells you if the article is research or clinically based	d. Hypothesis
_____	5. Statistical results from the study are explained	e. Variable
_____	6. A detailed background of previous studies	f. Analysis

Complete the following:

7. Evidence-based practice is:

8. Identify three valuable sources of nonresearch-based evidence.

9. A peer-reviewed article is:

10. A qualitative research study focuses on:

Copyright © 2019, Elsevier Inc. All Rights Reserved.

11. Provide an example of how a nurse integrates evidence into practice.

12. In the Quality Improvement model, what does PDSA stand for?

    P -

    D -

    S -

    A -

13. Provide at least one example of a patient outcome and measurement.

14. A randomized control trial (RCT) includes which of the following? Select all that apply.

    a. Subjects _____

    b. Experimental therapies _____

    c. A control group _____

    d. Subjective input from the researcher _____

    e. Analysis of the results _____

15. An evidence-based article includes which of the following? Select all that apply.

    a. An abstract _____

    b. The author's biography _____

    c. A literature review _____

    d. The study's design and methods _____

    e. The author's opinions about the subjects _____

    f. A conclusion relevant to the findings _____

16. Identify three of the competencies for evidence-based practice.

17. Sources for new scientific information are:

18. In a research study, the statistical analysis indicated a "p value" of 0.02. This is understood as being a good result.

    True _____ False _____

19. Two examples of comprehensive databases are:

20. Identify how evidence-based practice change can be communicated to others.

21. Root cause analysis is:

22. For the following study, identify each of the PICOT components:

    Over a 4-month period, the nursing staff on the unit is going to observe whether wound healing of pressure ulcers is improved if they are left open to air for 2 hours each day, rather than covered for 24 hours.

    P -

    I -

    C -

    O-

    T-

23. Identify three of the National Database of Nursing Quality Indicators (NDNQI).

24. Indicate at least two benefits from evidence-based practice.

25. A nursing sensitive outcome is:

26. The strongest evidence collection is found in Level _____ studies.

Select the best answer for each of the following questions:

27. A nurse recognizes which of the following as a sentinel event?
    1. An error is made and a medication dose is skipped.
    2. A wound infection is noted on a patient who has transferred from a nursing home.
    3. A patient is discharged within 72 hours of admission to the medical center.
    4. A hip replacement is performed on the wrong leg.

Copyright © 2019, Elsevier Inc. All Rights Reserved.

28. Which of the following is the best description of a case control study?
   1. A comparison of one group of subjects to another
   2. A focus on a subgroup with a known condition
   3. A prediction or explanation of phenomena
   4. A description of the responses to an independent variable

29. Which of the following is one of the skills that is embedded in the QSEN competency for evidence-based practice (EBP)?
   1. Value the need for ethical conduct of research and quality improvement
   2. Locate evidence reports related to clinical practice topics and guidelines
   3. Base individualized care plan on patient values, clinical expertise, and evidence
   4. Describe EBP to include components of research evidence and clinical expertise

STUDY GROUP QUESTIONS

- What is evidence-based practice?
- What is the seven-step process for evidence-based practice?
- How does a nurse become involved in the research process?
- What is PICO(T)?
- Where can reliable research-based data be found?
- What databases represent the scientific knowledge of health care?
- What types of evidence or studies are available for reference?
- How are evidence-based findings used in nursing practice?
- How are evidence-based changes communicated and evaluated?
- What is the relationship between evidence-based practice and quality improvement?
- What is the difference between evidence-based practice and research?

Copyright © 2019, Elsevier Inc. All Rights Reserved.

8 Critical Thinking

PRELIMINARY READING

Chapter 8, pp. 100–116

CASE STUDIES

1. You receive reports on your patient assignment for the day. You have six patients who require assessment and have orders for treatments and medications.
   a. How can you use critical thinking to approach this multiple patient assignment?

2. As a home care nurse, you have been assigned to visit a patient who requires dressing changes for a foot ulceration. When you arrive in the home, you see that the patient does not have any commercially packaged dressings or saline solution. You have used the last of your supplies, and the drive to the office will take more than 1 hour. The dressing that the patient has on her foot is saturated with purulent drainage.
   a. What options are available to you in this situation?
   b. What further investigation about the patient and her living situation may be necessary?

3. A patient, who has just been diagnosed with cancer, is being discharged to his home. The chemotherapy has altered his taste and reduced his appetite.
   a. Using critical thinking skills, what areas will you focus on for this patient?

CHAPTER REVIEW

Match the description/definition in Column A with the correct term in Column B.

	Column A	*Column B*
_____	1. Process of recalling an event to determine its meaning and purpose	a. Scientific method
_____	2. Series of clinical judgments that result in informal or formal diagnoses	b. Decision making
_____	3. End point of critical thinking that leads to problem resolution	c. Intuition
_____	4. Inner sensing that something is so	d. Diagnostic reasoning
_____	5. Process that moves from observable facts from an experience to a reasonable explanation of those facts	e. Reflection

Complete the following:

6. Identify one example of how critical thinking is used in each of the following steps of the nursing process:
   a. Assessment
   b. Nursing diagnosis
   c. Planning
   d. Implementation
   e. Evaluation

7. Identify the level of critical thinking demonstrated by each of the following:
   a. Trusting experts to have the right answers for every problem
   b. Analyzing and examining problems more independently
   c. Making choices without assistance and accepting accountability

Copyright © 2019, Elsevier Inc. All Rights Reserved.

8. Indicate the elements of the critical thinking model.

9. Identify the attitude of critical thinking demonstrated for each of the following:
   a. Performing a skill safely and effectively
   _____

   b. Questioning an order that appears incorrect
   _____

   c. Performing a systematic and thorough pain assessment _____

   d. Developing a unique way to teach the patient how to change a dressing _____

   e. Admitting to the nurse manager that a medication was given in error _____

10. Provide an example of how reflection could be used by the nurse in this scenario:
    The patient has had a colostomy and will need to learn self-care. The nurse has had many patients with new colostomies, some who have done well and others who have struggled to learn the care.

11. What are two useful tools for developing critical thinking skills?

12. Which of the following statements are accurate regarding critical thinking attitudes? Select all that apply.
    a. Risk-taking is not desirable in patient care. _____

    b. Using disciplined thinking reduces creativity. _____

    c. Perseverance can indicate that one is always looking for available resources. _____

    d. Personal feelings should not be allowed to influence delivery of care. _____

    e. All sides of each situation should be considered. _____

    f. Intuition should be used as a primary tool in determining patient care. _____

Select the best answer for each of the following questions:

13. In employing critical thinking, the first step that the nurse should take is:
    1. evaluation.
    2. decision making.
    3. self-regulation.
    4. interpretation.

14. Having worked for a number of years in the acute care environment, a nurse achieved the ability to use a complex level of critical thinking. The nurse:
    1. acts solely on his or her own opinions.
    2. trusts the experts to have the answers to problems.
    3. implements creative and innovative options.
    4. applies rules and principles the same way in every situation.

15. Clinical care experiences have recently begun for a student nurse. When beginning to work with patients, the student nurse implements critical thinking in practice by:
    1. asking for assistance if uncertain.
    2. sharing personal ideas with peers.
    3. acting on independent judgments.
    4. relying on standardized, textbook approaches.

16. A nurse has an extremely large patient assignment this evening and begins to feel overwhelmed. Of the following, what is the nurse's priority activity?
    1. Sharing his or her feelings with colleagues
    2. Calling the supervisor and asking for assistance
    3. Reviewing the overall assignment to get his or her bearings
    4. Moving immediately to provide patient care, starting with the room closest to the nurse's station

17. Orientation for new nurses begins. The instructor assembled information on critical thinking and nursing approaches. The instructor recognizes that critical thinkers in nursing:
    1. make quick, single-solution decisions.
    2. act on intuition instead of experience.
    3. review data in a organized manner.
    4. alter interventions for every circumstance.

18. A nurse is caring for a patient who is experiencing a respiratory disorder. Intuition is a part of the critical thinking process for the nurse. While caring for the patient, the nurse demonstrates intuition by:
    1. reviewing care with the patient in advance.
    2. observing communication patterns.
    3. establishing a nursing diagnosis.
    4. sensing that the patient is not doing as well as this morning.

Copyright © 2019, Elsevier Inc. All Rights Reserved.

19. Entering a room at 2:00 AM, a nurse notes that the patient is not in bed; the patient is sitting in the chair and states that she is having difficulty sleeping. Employing critical thinking, the nurse responds by:
    1. assisting the patient back into bed.
    2. asking more about the patient's sleep problem.
    3. positioning the patient and providing a warm blanket.
    4. obtaining an order for a hypnotic medication.

20. A nurse has a diverse patient assignment this evening. When reviewing the patients' conditions, the nurse determines that the first individual that should be seen is the patient:
    1. who is hypotensive.
    2. receiving a visit from a family member.
    3. being treated by the respiratory therapist.
    4. waiting for the effects of an analgesic that was given 5 minutes ago.

21. In using the critical thinking skill of self-regulation, a nurse will:
    1. be orderly in data collection.
    2. look at all situations objectively.
    3. use scientific and experiential knowledge.
    4. reflect on his or her own experiences and improve performance.

22. During the process of reflection, what is the most appropriate question for a nurse to ask himself or herself?
    1. "What could I have done differently?"
    2. "What's going on right now?"
    3. "How can the patient's status change?"
    4. "What should I do to communicate this information?"

23. A nurse believes that substance abuse is a serious problem with negative consequences for patients and families. The nurse, however, provides excellent care to a patient who is admitted with this problem. The nurse is displaying the critical thinking attitude of:
    1. integrity.
    2. fairness.
    3. discipline.
    4. perseverance.

24. In applying the concepts of critical thinking, the nurse demonstrates systematicity by:
    1. trusting his/her own reasoning processes.
    2. being organized and focused and working hard.
    3. reflecting on his/her own judgments.
    4. being tolerant of different patient viewpoints.

STUDY GROUP QUESTIONS

- How is critical thinking integrated into nursing practice?
- What attitudes are needed by a nurse in order to be a critical thinker?
- How are the competencies of critical thinking applied in clinical practice?
- Why is critical thinking important throughout the nursing process?

Copyright © 2019, Elsevier Inc. All Rights Reserved.

9 | Nursing Process

PRELIMINARY READING

Chapter 9, pp. 117–156

CASE STUDIES

1. Mr. B., a 47-year-old male patient, goes to the annual community health fair. During a routine blood pressure screening, it is determined that his blood pressure is significantly above normally expected levels.
   a. What additional assessment data should be obtained from the patient and family?
   b. What limitations exist in this situation for completing an assessment?

2. Mr. B. returns for a follow-up visit at the medical center's adult health clinic. Mr. B. is diagnosed with hypertension and an antihypertensive medication is prescribed, but he appears unsure about how and when he should take the prescription. He has no previous knowledge about hypertension or the medication. Mr. B. also says several times that his father died from a heart attack at 54 years old.
   a. Identify the relevant assessment data for this patient.
   b. Based upon this information, identify two nursing diagnoses.
   c. Based on the nursing diagnoses that were developed,
      (1) Identify one long-term or short-term goal for each diagnosis and at least one expected outcome for each goal.

Nursing diagnoses	Long-term or short-term goals	Expected outcomes
1.		
2.		

      (2) Identify two nursing interventions that may be appropriate in assisting the patient to achieve the expected outcomes and goals.

3. At his next visit to the adult health clinic, Mr. B. tells the nurse that he is taking the antihypertensive medication that was ordered by the physician "when he remembers." He says that he is trying to use the relaxation techniques that he was taught during his last visit, but he does not use them regularly.
   a. What nursing implementation methods should take priority at this time?
   b. What, if any, alterations need to be made in the original plan of care?

4. Mr. B. returns to the adult health clinic for evaluation of his status. His blood pressure is lower than before but remains slightly above normal limits. He exercises once or twice a week, and states that this is making him feel better. Mr. B. shows the nurse a calendar where he has marked down the times for taking his medication. Mr. B. relates that he has been trying very hard to use the relaxation techniques when he starts to feel anxious or overwhelmed. He identifies that he cannot control all of his "destiny," but he is trying to do things that may help him avoid what happened to his father.
   a. In accordance with previously identified outcomes, what nursing evaluation may be made on this patient's status?
   b. What areas, if any, may require reassessment?

5. A 4-year-old girl is newly diagnosed with diabetes mellitus. You are going to be working with the family to help them to adjust to the treatment regimen.
   a. What assessment data are important to collect from the child and family?
   b. Identify a possible nursing diagnosis for the child or the family related to the new diagnosis.

Copyright © 2019, Elsevier Inc. All Rights Reserved.

Match the description/definition in Column A with the correct term in Column B.

Column A

_____ 1. Unintended effect of a medication, diagnostic test, or intervention

_____ 2. Observations or measurements made by the nurse during assessment

_____ 3. Comparing data with another source to determine accuracy and relevancy

_____ 4. Identifies relationships between nursing diagnoses and interventions

_____ 5. Clinical judgment about patient responses to health problems or life processes

_____ 6. Information obtained through the senses

_____ 7. Activities performed in the course of a normal day

_____ 8. Support for why a specific nursing action is chosen

_____ 9. Interpretation of cues

_____ 10. Information verbally provided by the patient

Column B

a. Subjective data

b. ADLs

c. Adverse reaction

d. Concept map

e. Nursing diagnosis

f. Cue

g. Objective data

h. Scientific rationale

i. Inference

j. Validation

Complete the following:

11. The three phases of an interview are:

12. Based on the following data clusters, identify possible nursing diagnoses:
    a. Abdominal pain, three loose liquid stools per day, hyperactive bowel sounds:
    b. Fatigue, weakness, tachycardia, and dyspnea upon activity:

13. Identify at least one goal or expected outcome and one nursing intervention for the following nursing diagnoses:
    a. *Lack of knowledge related to the need for postoperative care at home*
    Goal:

    Expected outcome:

    Nursing intervention:

b. *Constipation related to lack of physical activity*
Goal:

Expected outcome:

Nursing intervention:

c. *Danger of personal injury associated with episodes of dizziness*
Goal:

Expected outcome:

Nursing intervention:

14. Identify whether the following are examples of cognitive, interpersonal, or psychomotor skills in patient care:
    a. Preparing and administering an injection
    b. Completing a health history
    c. Providing emotional support to a family member
    d. Changing a surgical dressing
    e. Recognizing the patient's need for nutritional instruction

Copyright © 2019, Elsevier Inc. All Rights Reserved.

15. Before implementing standing orders, the nurse should check:

16. The steps of the implementation phase of the nursing process are:

17. During interactions with a patient, a nurse gathers more data and identifies a new patient need. The nurse modifies the plan of care by:

18. A patient with diabetes mellitus goes to the outpatient center for care. There is a written plan for diet counseling, medication, and follow-up care. These specific procedures are termed a(n) _____ for care.

19. An example of an indirect nursing intervention is:

20. Identify all of the following that typically may be delegated to unlicensed assistive personnel:

    a. Skin care _____

    b. Tracheostomy care _____

    c. Hygienic care _____

    d. Personal grooming _____

    e. Urinary catheterization _____

    f. Administration of IV medications _____

    g. Assistance with ambulation _____

21. Specify how the wording of the following patient outcome statements may be improved according to the SMART acronym:
    a. Erythema will be less noticeable.
    b. Pulse rate will be normal.
    c. Patient's calorie intake will increase.
    d. Wound will be healed shortly.
    e. Patient will ambulate in the hospital.

22. Identify at least three ways to create a good environment for an interview with a patient.

23. Indicate whether the following data are subjective or objective:
    a. "I feel tired."
    b. BP 124/64
    c. Pain level of 5 on a scale of 10
    d. Diaphoresis
    e. Wound edges dry and intact

24. What information can be found in a patient's medical record?

25. How would the following data be validated by the nurse?
    a. Patient states that he is fatigued.
    b. The pressure ulcer appears larger.

26. Provide examples of how the nurse can implement each of the following in the plan of care:
    a. Direct care
    b. Counseling
    c. Teaching
    d. Controlling adverse reactions

27. What are the steps in the evaluation process?

28. Provide an example of how the nurse can determine the patient's cultural needs or preferences.

29. For a nursing diagnosis related to a patient's inability to feed herself, indicate two interventions that the nurse can implement to assist the patient.

30. The Nurse Practice Acts in all states require accurate data collection and recording as independent functions essential to the role of a professional nurse.

    True _____ False _____

31. Provide an example of what the nurse would say when back-channeling.

32. When the nurse does not know how to perform a procedure, the appropriate actions are to:

Copyright © 2019, Elsevier Inc. All Rights Reserved.

33. A *care bundle* is:

34. The health care team at the local clinic needs the medical treatment history from the time the patient was hospitalized. What procedure should be followed to obtain this information?

35. How should the nurse clarify or validate the following patient statements?
    a. "I'm really tired in the afternoon."
    b. "I have trouble sticking to a diet."
    c. "I've noticed that my urine is really dark and I don't go to the bathroom as often as I used to."
    d. "I have a hard time doing what I used to because of the muscle and joint pain."

Select the best answer for each of the following questions:

36. A new graduate is preparing to work with patients on a medical unit. The nursing process is applied as a:
    1. method for processing the care of many patients.
    2. tool for diagnosing and treating patients' health problems.
    3. guideline for determining the nurse's accountability in patient care.
    4. logical, problem-solving approach to providing patient care.

37. Upon admission, the nurse begins to assess the patient. The patient appears uncomfortable, stating that she has severe abdominal pain. The nurse should:
    1. inquire specifically about the discomfort.
    2. let the patient rest, returning later to complete the assessment.
    3. perform a complete physical examination immediately.
    4. ask the family about the patient's health history.

38. The following nursing diagnoses are proposed for patients on the medical unit. The diagnostic statement that contains all of the necessary components is:
    1. *reduced oxygenation associated with excessive lung secretions.*
    2. *insufficient nutrition related to medical treatment.*
    3. *experiencing grief.*
    4. *pain from abdominal surgery.*

39. In reviewing the nursing diagnoses written by a new staff member, a supervisor identifies which of the following as a correctly written nursing diagnosis?
    1. *Altered respiratory function related to abnormal blood gases*
    2. *Urinary infection related to long-term catheterization*
    3. *Insufficient understanding of the need for cardiac monitoring*
    4. *Pain from severe arthritis in finger joints*

40. A nurse is working with a patient who has the following symptoms: dyspnea, ankle edema, weight gain, abdominal distention, hypertension. The nursing diagnosis that is most appropriate for these signs and symptoms is:
    1. *insufficient tissue oxygenation.*
    2. *altered body image.*
    3. *altered respiratory function.*
    4. *increased fluid volume.*

41. A patient is to have abdominal surgery tomorrow. The nurse determines that an outcome for this patient that meets the necessary criteria is:
    1. patient will be repositioned every 2 hours.
    2. patient will express fears about surgery.
    3. patient will achieve normal elimination pattern before discharge.
    4. patient will perform active range-of-motion exercises every 2 hours while in bed.

42. There are a number of activities that are to be performed by a nurse during a clinical shift. In deciding to perform a nurse-initiated intervention, the nurse:
    1. administers oral medications.
    2. orders laboratory tests.
    3. changes a sterile dressing.
    4. teaches newborn hygienic care.

43. A nurse implements a preventive nursing action when:
    1. immunizing patients.
    2. assisting with hygienic care.
    3. inserting a urinary catheter.
    4. providing crisis intervention counseling.

44. A nurse has been working with a patient in the rehabilitative facility for 2 weeks. The nurse is in the process of evaluating the patient's progress. During the evaluation phase, the nurse recognizes that:
    1. nursing diagnoses always remain the same.
    2. time frames for patient outcomes may be adjusted.
    3. evaluative skills differ greatly from those for patient assessment.
    4. the number of nursing diagnoses and outcomes is most important.

Copyright © 2019, Elsevier Inc. All Rights Reserved.

45. An expected outcome for a patient is the following: "Pulse will remain below 120 beats per minute during exercise." If the patient's pulse rate exceeds 120 beats per minute one of every three exercise periods, the nurse appropriately evaluates the patient's goal attainment as:
   1. patient has achieved desired behavior.
   2. patient requires further evaluation of progress.
   3. patient's response indicates need for elimination of exercise.
   4. patient does not comply with therapeutic regimen.

46. The nurse is caring for a patient who has been medically stable. During the change-of-shift report, the nurse is informed that the patient is experiencing a slight arrhythmia. To avoid complications during the implementation of care, the nurse plans to first:
   1. evaluate the patient's vital signs.
   2. ask about the patient's previous diagnoses.
   3. contact the physician immediately.
   4. tell the nursing assistant to perform the usual care for the patient.

47. For a patient in the acute care facility, a nurse identifies several interventions. The statement that best communicates the specific nursing intervention to be performed is:
   1. assist with exercises.
   2. take the patient's vital signs.
   3. refer the patient to a therapist.
   4. provide 30 mL of water with the nasogastric tube feedings every 4 hours.

48. The nurse is working with a patient who has diabetes mellitus. The nursing diagnosis is *reduced fluid volume related to diuresis*. An appropriate patient outcome, based on this nursing diagnosis, is:
   1. patient will have an increased urinary output.
   2. patient will decrease the amount of fluid intake during a 24-hour period.
   3. patient will demonstrate a decrease in edema in the lower extremities.
   4. patient will have palpable peripheral pulses and good capillary refill.

49. A nurse is working with a patient who is experiencing abnormal breath sounds and thick secretions. The nurse identifies a nursing diagnosis of:
   1. *decreased body fluid volume.*
   2. *insufficient airway clearance.*
   3. *potential for altered mucous membranes.*
   4. *ineffective respiratory response.*

50. In completing a health history, a nurse obtains from the patient psychosocial information that includes:
   1. the reason for seeking health care.
   2. past health problems.
   3. the primary language spoken.
   4. physical safety status.

51. A patient tells the nurse that she feels she may not be using the crutches correctly when ambulating. The best way for the nurse to validate this information is to:
   1. ask the family about the patient's ambulation.
   2. ask the physician how the patient was taught.
   3. discuss the problem with the other staff members.
   4. observe the patient using the crutches.

52. An example of the most appropriately written nursing diagnosis is:
   1. *discomfort related to surgery.*
   2. *shortness of breath related to immobility.*
   3. *anxiety related to insufficient knowledge about cardiac monitoring.*
   4. *recurrent infection related to improper catheterization procedure.*

53. In determining which of the following patients on the medical unit to visit first, a nurse selects the patient with which of the following diagnoses?
   1. *Increased nutritional intake*
   2. *Insufficient tissue oxygenation*
   3. *Lack of knowledge regarding home care resources*
   4. *Reduction in physical mobility*

54. An example of a physician-initiated intervention is:
   1. teaching a patient about the therapeutic diet.
   2. assessing a patient's skin.
   3. providing emotional support.
   4. preparing a patient for a diagnostic test.

55. The new nurse seeks the expertise of the dietician in the medical center. This is an example of:
   1. consultation.
   2. validation.
   3. inference.
   4. mapping.

56. Which of the following is the most appropriate patient outcome statement?
   1. Patient will be fed three times each day.
   2. Patient will be free of disease.
   3. Patient will learn about the wound care.
   4. Patient will identify times to contact the provider after discharge.

STUDY GROUP QUESTIONS

- What is involved in patient assessment, and what priorities does a nurse have in completing an assessment?
- How does the patient assessment fit into the nursing process?
- Why does an error in the assessment phase influence the remaining implementation of the process, and how can a nurse avoid errors?
- What methods may be used to obtain patient data, and what type of data is obtained with each method?
- What is involved in a patient interview?

29

Copyright © 2019, Elsevier Inc. All Rights Reserved.

- How can a nurse optimize the environment for a patient interview?
- How can a nurse use different communication strategies to obtain data during patient assessment?
- What is a nursing diagnosis?
- What are the components of a nursing diagnosis?
- How are actual and potential nursing diagnoses different?
- How are medical and nursing diagnoses different?
- What errors are possible in formulating nursing diagnoses, and how may they be avoided?
- Which nursing diagnoses become priorities in planning patient care?
- How are long-term and short-term goals different from each other?
- How are goals and expected outcomes different from each other?
- What are the guidelines for formulating goals and outcomes?
- How is the SMART acronym used for writing goals and expected outcomes?
- In selecting nursing interventions, what are three essential nurse competencies?
- How are the three types of nursing interventions different from one another?
- What factors should be considered when selecting nursing interventions?
- What is the purpose of the care plan, and what types are available for use?

- How does a critical pathway differ from a "traditional" care plan?
- How does the consultation process begin, and who and what may be involved in the process?
- What is the focus of the implementation phase of the nursing process?
- What are standing orders and protocols, and how are they used in patient care situations?
- What are the five preparatory nursing activities that are completed before implementing the care plan?
- What are the nursing implementation methods?
- How is nursing implementation communicated to other members of the health care team?
- How is evaluation incorporated into the nursing process?
- How is evaluation used in patient situations and in nursing practice and health care delivery settings?
- What circumstances would lead to a modification of a care plan?

STUDY CHART

Create a study chart to compare the *Steps of the Nursing Process* that identifies the different activities involved in each step.

Create a *Concept Map* for one of the case studies in this chapter.

Copyright © 2019, Elsevier Inc. All Rights Reserved.

10 Informatics and Documentation

PRELIMINARY READING

Chapter 10, pp. 157–177

CASE STUDIES

1. Mrs. Q. has just been transferred to her room from the postanesthesia care unit (PACU) after right hip replacement surgery. She was accompanied by a nurse from PACU. Vital signs were taken upon transfer and found to be within expected limits. A dressing is in place on the patient's right hip. Mrs. Q. does not appear to be having any difficulty at the moment.
   a. What information should be provided by the PACU nurse in the hand-off report to the primary nurse on the surgical unit when Mrs. Q. is transferred to her room?
   b. What additional information may Mrs. Q.'s primary nurse want to obtain from the PACU nurse?

2. The primary nurse begins to plan and provide care for Mrs. Q. Upon entering the patient's room, Mrs. Q. is found to be grimacing and moaning in pain. She says that she is having intense pain in her right hip area. The dressing to her hip is dry and intact. Mrs. Q. says that she does not want to move because it really hurts. The primary nurse helps Mrs. Q. to get into a more comfortable position and begins to prepare the pain medication ordered by the physician. The primary nurse administers the pain medication, and, after approximately one-half hour, Mrs. Q. states that the pain has been reduced. Using the SOAP or DAR method, document the nursing interaction with Mrs. Q.

3. Mr. W. has just been diagnosed with type 1 diabetes mellitus and needs to learn how to self-administer his insulin injections.
   a. What information should be included in the patient record regarding the teaching provided to Mr. W. on the self-injection of insulin?

CHAPTER REVIEW

Match the description/definition in Column A with the correct term in Column B.

	Column A	Column B
_____	1. An oral or written exchange of information between health care providers	a. Record
_____	2. Information about patients provided only to appropriate personnel	b. POMR
_____	3. Permanent communication with patient's health care management	c. Acuity level
_____	4. Structured method of documentation with emphasis on the patient's problems	d. Report
_____	5. A classification used to compare one or more patients to another group of patients.	e. Confidentiality

Copyright © 2019, Elsevier Inc. All Rights Reserved.

Complete the following:

6. The following are guidelines for written documentation. Indicate the correct action to be taken by the nurse for each guideline.
   a. Never erase entries or use correction fluid, and never use pencil.
   b. Do not write retaliatory or critical comments about patients.
   c. Avoid using generalized, empty phrases.
   d. Do not cross out errors.
   e. Do not leave blank spaces.
   f. Do not speculate or guess.
   g. Do not record: "Physician made error."
   h. Never record or chart for someone else.
   i. Do not wait until the end of shift to record important information.

7. a. HIPAA (Health Insurance Portability and Accountability Act of 1996) requires providers to notify patients of privacy policies.

   True _____ False _____

   b. Incident or occurrence reports should be documented in the patient's medical record in the nurses' narrative notes section.

   True _____ False _____

   c. Poor written and verbal communication has been one of the top 10 reasons for sentinel events.

   True _____ False _____

   d. Patients have the right to request copies of their medical records and read the information.

   True _____ False _____

8. Standards for health care agencies and documentation are set by the:

9. For each of the following, identify an example of how the patient record is used:
   a. Communication:
   b. Finance:
   c. Education:
   d. Research:
   e. Auditing/monitoring:

10. Provide an example of a malpractice issue related to charting:

11. Identify the five characteristics of quality documentation:

12. Subjective statements made by the patient are best documented by:

13. Demonstrate how a student nurse should sign a written patient record:

14. Identify what is wrong with the following notations and how they can be corrected:
    a. "Ate some breakfast."
    b. "Voided an adequate amount."
    c. "Provided wound care qd."

15. For telephone reports, identify what the SBAR acronym represents and give an example of each area:
    S:
    B:
    A:
    R:

16. Provide two items that should be included in a discharge summary:

17. Home care documentation is completed both for quality control and as the basis for:

18. Completion of narrative notes only when there are abnormal patient findings is part of the concept of:

19. What are the purposes and advantages of nursing informatics?

20. Identify at least two ways in which electronic records are safeguarded for privacy and security:

21. Identify the four concepts included in informatics:

Copyright © 2019, Elsevier Inc. All Rights Reserved.

22. Which of the following are the correct nursing actions for a telephone order? Select all that apply.

    a. Identifying that Mr. J. is in Room 212. _____

    b. Asking the physician to repeat the medication order for Mr. J. four times. _____

    c. Checking that 40 mg of the drug is the amount that should be given. _____

    d. Identifying "TO" (telephone order) in the nurse's notes. _____

    e. Asking another nurse to call the physician back to verify the order. _____

    f. Having Mr. J.'s doctor cosign the order within 24 hours. _____

23. What information is usually available to nurses on a clinical information system (CIS)?

24. A problem-oriented medical record includes which of the following? Select all that apply.

    a. Progress notes _____

    b. Narrative notes _____

    c. Database _____

    d. Problem list _____

    e. Incident reports _____

    f. Care plan _____

25. As a student nurse, what information should be left off written materials that are prepared for class?

26. Identify the errors in the following documentation example:
    Patient says she feels ok. 140/82, 88, 14. Gained a little weight. Complained about her doctor. Says she didn't eat much breakfast today.

27. The patient is admitted to the medical center with a Stage IV pressure ulcer. The nurse recognizes the implications of this finding.
    a. This specific finding is classified as a: _____.

    b. What does the nurse need to document?

28. Which of the following are correct statements regarding standardized care plans? Select all that apply.

    a. They facilitate safe and consistent care for an identified problem. _____

    b. They replace the need for nursing decision-making and judgments. _____

    c. The same interventions, goals, and outcomes are used for all patients. _____

    d. Evidence-based guidelines are able to be accessed. _____

    e. Institutional standards may be described. _____

    f. They are not used to conduct quality improvement audits. _____

29. Which of the following require occurrence/incident reports? Select all that apply.
    a. A patient's visitor is hit by a portable x-ray machine. _____

    b. The patient falls out of bed. _____

    c. A nurse documents in the wrong record. _____

    d. The patient refuses a medication. _____

    e. A nurse sticks herself with a needle. _____

    f. An inaccurate medication dosage is administered. _____

Select the best answer for each of the following questions:

30. A nurse is working in a facility that uses computerized documentation of patient information. To maintain patient confidentiality with the use of computerized documentation, the nurse should:
    1. delete any and all errors made in the record.
    2. only give his or her password to other nurses working with the patient.
    3. log off the file or computer when not using the terminal.
    4. remove sensitive patient information, such as communicable diseases, from the record.

31. The nurses on a medical unit in an acute care facility are meeting to select a documentation format to use. They recognize that less fragmentation of patient data will occur if they implement:
    1. source records.
    2. focus charting.
    3. charting by exception.
    4. critical pathways.

33

Copyright © 2019, Elsevier Inc. All Rights Reserved.

32. While caring for a patient on the surgical unit, a nurse notes that the patient's blood pressure has dropped significantly since the last measurement. The nurse shares this information immediately with the health care provider in a(n):
   1. flow sheet record.
   2. incident report.
   3. telephone report.
   4. change-of-shift report.

33. Documentation of patient care is reviewed during the orientation to the facility. The new graduate nurse understands that the method for written documentation that is acceptable is:
   1. using red ink to make entries on patients' charts.
   2. charting all of the patient care at the end of the shift.
   3. beginning each entry with the time of the treatment or observation.
   4. leaving space at the end of the notations to allow for additional documentation.

34. A nurse is caring for a patient who has had abdominal surgery. Accurate and complete documentation of the care provided by the nurse is evident by the following notation:
   1. "Vital signs taken."
   2. "Tylenol with codeine given for pain."
   3. "Provided adequate amount of fluid."
   4. "10 AM - IV fluids increased to 100 mL per hour according to protocol."

35. A nurse is involved in patient care in an agency that uses military time for documentation. Which of the following represents 4:00 PM?
   1. 0400
   2. 0800
   3. 1400
   4. 1600

36. An example of the use of a clinical decision support system (CDSS) is:
   1. access to patient's lab reports.
   2. direct input to the medical orders by the health care provider.
   3. problem-oriented recording.
   4. an alert for incorrect drug dosages.

37. An appropriate action by a student nurse is demonstrated by:
   1. accessing records of other students' patients.
   2. writing the patient's name and room number on assignments.
   3. copying patient records for review and preparation of care plans.
   4. reading the patient's record in preparation for clinical care.

38. A nurse enters a patient's room and discovers a yellow pill on the bed under the patient's pillow. The patient receives Lasix 40 mg daily. Which of the following notations is appropriate to include on an incident or occurrence report?
   1. "Patient refused to take Lasix at 10 AM."
   2. "Yellow pill found on bed under pillow."
   3. "Lasix not administered by primary nurse."
   4. "Patient did not receive 10 AM diuretic."

39. Which of the following statements made by a new staff nurse during change-of-shift report requires correction?
   1. "The patient is really uncooperative about doing his stoma care."
   2. "Oxygen is needed after ambulation. This is a change in priorities."
   3. "Ms. Q is a 62-year-old with diabetes mellitus."
   4. "The abdominal surgical wound is healing slowly, with no drainage noted."

STUDY GROUP QUESTIONS

- What is the purpose of documentation and reporting?
- What are the legal guidelines for documentation?
- How do the guidelines influence nursing documentation and reporting?
- What methods are available for documentation of patient data?
- How do the different types of documentation (for example, SOAP, DAR, and narrative) compare with one another?
- How does written documentation compare with computerized systems, and what are the advantages and disadvantages of each method?
- What types of forms are used for patient documentation?
- How does patient documentation change in different health care settings?
- What information is necessary when doing change-of-shift, telephone, transfer, and incident reports?
- What role does informatics play in heath care?
- How do nurses use information systems?
- What safety measures need to be taken by nurses when accessing electronic records?
- What type of patient information is accessible on electronic systems?

Copyright © 2019, Elsevier Inc. All Rights Reserved.

11 Communication

Chapter 11, pp. 178–200

CASE STUDIES

1. For the following patient situations, identify the communication techniques that may be most effective in establishing a nurse-patient relationship:
   a. An older adult patient who has a moderate hearing impairment
   b. The Russian-speaking parents of a young child who has been taken into the emergency department after a bicycle accident
   c. A young adult patient who is blind and requires daily insulin injections
   d. A 60-year-old Hispanic woman who will be having her first internal pelvic examination
   e. A 45-year-old patient on a ventilator
   f. A 65-year-old man who has just been diagnosed with cancer and is very anxious

2. You are working with a patient who appears to have literacy issues. There is a need to instruct the patient about the medical diagnosis.
   a. What strategies should you use to assist the patient to understand the diagnosis and treatment plan?

CHAPTER REVIEW

Match the description/definition in Column A with the correct term in Column B.

	Column A	Column B
_____	1. Person who initiates interpersonal communication	a. Therapeutic communication
_____	2. Information sent or expressed by the sender	b. Metacommunication
_____	3. Means of conveying messages	c. Sender
_____	4. Person to whom the message is sent	d. Intonation
_____	5. Indicates whether the meaning of the sender's message was received	e. Feedback
_____	6. Tone of the speaker's voice that may affect a message's meaning	f. Channels
_____	7. A message within a message that conveys a sender's attitude toward the self and toward the listener	g. Message
_____	8. Development of a working, functional relationship by the nurse with the patient, fulfilling the purposes of the nursing process	h. Receiver

Complete the following:

9. Determine what level of communication the following examples illustrate:
   a. Speaking to a community group about a health-related topic
   b. "He looks uncomfortable, and I want to show him that I'm concerned about his discomfort."
   c. Talking to oneself

10. Provide an example of how compassion fatigue may develop.

35

11. Individuals maintain distances between themselves during interactions. Identify the zone (Intimate, Personal, Social, or Public) that is being used in each of the following examples:
   a. Speaking to a group of students in a classroom

   _____

   b. Conducting a small group therapy session

   _____

   c. Performing a physical examination _____

   d. Making patient rounds with a physician

   _____

   e. Changing a wound dressing _____

   f. Testifying at a hearing _____

   g. Completing a change-of-shift report _____

12. For an older adult with impaired communication, identify the appropriate communication techniques. Select all that apply:
   a. Maintaining a quiet environment that is free of

   background noise _____

   b. Shifting from subject to subject during the conversation _____

   c. Letting the person know if you are having difficulty understanding him or her _____

   d. Using explorative questions to facilitate conversation _____

   e. Using long sentences to explain subject matter

   _____

13. The following are examples of inappropriate communication by a nurse. Specify an effective strategy that should be used to correct the situation:
   a. Calling the patient "Honey"

   b. Reporting to a nursing colleague about the "gallbladder in room 214"

   c. Talking about a patient to other nurses in the elevator

   d. Running into a patient's room to administer medications and then leaving immediately

   e. Informing a patient that the physician will be performing an abdominal hysterectomy and that she should expect a midline incision of approximately 10 centimeters

   f. Speaking to a patient while chewing gum

14. For the following examples, identify a question that the nurse could ask that would be more appropriate and would obtain better information from the patient:
   a. "You're feeling okay today, right?"

   b. "You don't take any medication at home, do you?"

   c. "Are you having any lymphedema?"

   d. "The physician will be doing a paracentesis today. He said he explained it to you."

   e. "You really don't seem to understand how serious your condition is!"

   f. "Why aren't you sticking with the prescribed diet?"

15. Identify the communication strategy that is being used for each of the following examples:
   a. Sitting with a patient who is crying

   b. Showing interest in the patient who is discussing concerns or sharing family information

   c. Saying "The test will take about 15 minutes to complete and you will be lying flat on the examination table."

   d. Asking the patient to verify the meaning of statements made

   e. Directing the attention of the patient to a particular idea in the discussion

16. For the patient who has aphasia and difficulty speaking or understanding, identify at least two nursing interventions to promote communication with the patient.

17. Nurses on a medical unit are discussing issues related to their work schedules. Identify the examples of positive responses:
   a. "There's nothing we can do about the staffing

   situation." _____

   b. "Don't talk to me like that!" _____

   c. "What do you think we can do to improve this

   situation?" _____

   d. "I want to hear what your concerns are." _____

Copyright © 2019, Elsevier Inc. All Rights Reserved.

18. A nurse takes into account cultural considerations when communicating with patients. Identify appropriate actions for the nurse to take to promote therapeutic communication.

19. For the acronym AIDET®, identify the skills for successful communication.
    A:
    I:
    D:
    E:
    T:

20. Identify the nursing actions/responses that occur during the Orientation Phase of the Helping Relationship. Select all that apply:
    a. Achieving a smooth transition for the patient to other caregivers as needed _____
    b. Providing information needed to understand and change behavior _____
    c. Reviewing available data, including the medical and nursing history _____
    d. Expecting the patient to test your competence and commitment _____
    e. Setting the tone for the relationship by adopting a warm, empathetic, caring manner _____
    f. Prioritizing patient problems and identifying patient goals _____

21. Rose is a new nurse on the cardiac unit. Her new colleagues, who have worked there for many years, do not help her and say things like "Didn't you learn that in school?" This is an example of:

22. Identify three physiological alterations that could influence communication for the patient:

23. How does communication influence collaboration and patient safety?

24. What is going on in the photo below that may interfere with communication between the nurse and the patient?

25. Which of the following characteristics are risks for violent behavior? Select all that apply:
    a. Over 65 years of age _____
    b. Female _____
    c. Admitted through the emergency department _____
    d. Has a history of violent behavior _____
    e. Has dementia _____

Select the best answer for each of the following questions:

26. A patient tells a nurse that he feels anxious and afraid. The nurse responds by saying, "I will stay here with you." The nurse is using the principle of effective communication known as:
    1. empathy.
    2. courtesy.
    3. presence.
    4. encouragement.

27. A patient states that he believes he may have cancer. The nurse tells him, "I wouldn't be concerned. I'm sure that the tests will be negative." The response by the nurse is demonstrating the use of a nontherapeutic response of:
    1. assertiveness.
    2. false reassurance.
    3. professional opinion.
    4. hope and encouragement.

28. A nurse is assigned to a young adult male patient. Gender sensitivity is demonstrated when the nurse:
    1. uses sexual innuendo.
    2. engages in gender-oriented joking.
    3. stereotypes male and female roles.
    4. uses direct and indirect communication appropriately.

Copyright © 2019, Elsevier Inc. All Rights Reserved.

29. A patient regularly visits a medical clinic. A nurse establishes a helping relationship with the patient. During the working phase of a helping relationship, the nurse:
   1. encourages and helps the patient to set goals.
   2. reminisces about the relationship with the patient.
   3. anticipates health concerns or issues.
   4. identifies a location for the interaction.

30. A nurse is interviewing a patient who is in the outpatient area. The nurse uses paraphrasing communication with the statement:
   1. "This is your blood pressure medication. It will help to lower your blood pressure to the level where it should be."
   2. "Do you mean that the pain comes and goes when you walk?"
   3. "I would like to return to our discussion about your family."
   4. "If I understand you correctly, you are primarily concerned about your dizzy spells."

31. A patient tells a nurse that there are other people in the room who are watching her from under the bed. The nurse employs therapeutic communication when he or she:
   1. identifies that there are no people under the bed.
   2. tells the patient that he or she will help look for the other people.
   3. asks the patient why other people are watching her.
   4. reassures the patient that he or she will tell the people to go away.

32. While speaking with a female patient, a nurse notes that she is frowning. The nurse wants to find out about possible concerns by:
   1. asking why the patient is unhappy.
   2. telling the patient that everything is fine.
   3. identifying that the patient is frowning.
   4. asking if the patient is angry about the health care problem.

33. A patient's condition has deteriorated, and he has been transferred to the intensive care unit. The roommate asks the nurse what is wrong with the patient. The nurse should respond to the roommate by stating:
   1. "The patient's condition is no concern of yours."
   2. "Everything is fine. Don't worry. He'll be okay."
   3. "I recognize your interest in the patient, but I cannot share personal information with you without his permission."
   4. "Your roommate's condition worsened overnight, and he had to be moved to the intensive care unit for observation."

34. A patient is experiencing aphasia as a result of a CVA (cerebrovascular accident, or stroke). To promote communication, a nurse plans to:
   1. speak louder.
   2. use more questions.
   3. use visual clues, such as pictures and gestures.
   4. refer to a speech therapist to communicate with the patient.

35. A patient is talking endlessly about problems in the past with arthritic pain, but the nurse needs to get specific information for the admission assessment. The nurse's best response is:
   1. "You seem to have had difficulty managing the arthritis. What are you doing now for the pain?"
   2. "You can tell me more at another time. We need to move on to other information now."
   3. "You've given me a lot of information, but I have to ask you something else."
   4. "Are you taking medication for the arthritis?"

36. A nurse enters a room and finds the patient crying. The best action by the nurse is to:
   1. ask the patient why he or she is crying.
   2. tell the patient that things will get better.
   3. let the patient know that you will come back later.
   4. sit quietly with the patient.

37. A patient has a visual impairment. In communicating with this patient, a nurse should:
   1. use flash cards.
   2. use simple sentences.
   3. caution the patient before any physical contact.
   4. speak very loudly and slowly.

38. A nurse tells the patient's family that recovery may be "difficult." With the use of this word, there may be an issue with:
   1. pacing.
   2. clarity.
   3. relevance.
   4. connotation.

39. The patient appears to be very stressed and tells the nurse that he is having a hard time managing. The nurse replies by saying, "It sounds like you are feeling overwhelmed." This is an example of:
   1. trust.
   2. empathy.
   3. providing information.
   4. automatic response.

Copyright © 2019, Elsevier Inc. All Rights Reserved.

40. A nurse is working with a preschool-age child. An appropriate communication technique to use with an individual in this age group is to:
    1. speak loudly and forcibly.
    2. communicate directly with the parents to determine the child's needs.
    3. sit or kneel down to be on the same level as the child.
    4. use medical terms when speaking with the parents so the child will not understand.

41. A patient's blood sample was dropped on its way to the lab. The patient asks the nurse why blood needs to be drawn again for the same test. The nurse's best response is:
    1. "One of the vials was dropped and broken by mistake. We will make sure that this sample gets to the lab safely."
    2. "We just have to do the test again."
    3. "Someone didn't do their job right the first time."
    4. "This kind of thing happens. It won't take long."

42. Which one of the following medications has the greatest potential to influence patient communication?
    1. Diuretics
    2. Antipsychotics
    3. Anticholinergics
    4. Antipyretics

43. A nurse is evaluating communication skills used during an interaction with a newly admitted patient. Of the statements made, the nurse responded therapeutically with:
    1. "Why aren't you able to keep taking the prescribed medications?"
    2. "We need to move quickly through the rest of the interview because it will be time for your therapy."
    3. "I can understand why you don't like that physician. I think you need to find another one."
    4. "I noticed that you didn't eat any of the lunch. Is there something that is bothering you?"

STUDY GROUP QUESTIONS

- What is therapeutic communication?
- What are the basic elements of communication?
- How do nurses and patients communicate verbally and nonverbally?
- What factors may influence communication?
- How can a patient's physical, psychosocial, and developmental status influence communication with the nurse?
- How is a helping relationship established with a patient?
- What are the principles/techniques of effective communication?
- How are these principles/techniques used by a nurse in a caring relationship?
- How is communication used within the steps of the nursing process?
- What are some of the barriers to effective communication, and how can they be overcome by the nurse?

STUDY CHART

Create a study chart to compare the *Components of Verbal and Nonverbal Communication* that identifies how each may influence the nurse-patient interaction (e.g., intonation).

Copyright © 2019, Elsevier Inc. All Rights Reserved.

12 Patient Education

PRELIMINARY READING

Chapter 12, pp. 201–220

CASE STUDIES

1. Your patient is a 47-year-old married woman who has gone to the medical clinic for evaluation. She has been diagnosed with hypertension and placed on an antihypertensive medication. She has no previous knowledge or experience with the diagnosis or the medication. There is a family history of coronary disease; her father died of a heart attack at 54 years old.
   a. What information about the patient may affect her motivation to learn?
   b. Formulate a teaching plan for the patient that includes goals and teaching strategies.

2. You are a nurse in a pediatrician's office. An 8-year-old boy has just been diagnosed with diabetes mellitus. His parents are very concerned about what this means for their son.
   a. What general information will the family need?
   b. How will you adapt your teaching for your 8-year-old patient?

3. You will give a presentation tomorrow to a small group of patients.
   a. What do you need to take into consideration when preparing the setting for the teaching session?

CHAPTER REVIEW

Match the description/definition in Column A with the correct term in Column B.

	Column A	Column B
_____	1. Expression of feelings, attitudes, opinions, and values	a. Cognitive learning
_____	2. Mental state that allows for focus and comprehension of material	b. Motivation
_____	3. Acquiring skills	c. Attentional set
_____	4. Intellectual behaviors, including knowledge and understanding	d. Affective learning
_____	5. An internal state that helps arouse, direct, and sustain human behavior	e. Return demonstration
_____	6. Completion of a procedure to show competence	f. Psychomotor learning

Complete the following:

7. a. What are the six aspects of the ACCESS model?

   b. What are the components of the ASSURE model?

   c. When would these models be used?

8. A mild level of anxiety may motivate learning.

   True _____ False _____

9. From the following, select the appropriate topics for health education related to health maintenance and promotion and illness prevention. Select all that apply:

   a. First aid _____

   b. Occupational therapy _____

   c. Implications of noncompliance with therapy _____

   d. Hygiene _____

   e. Origin of symptoms _____

   f. Immunizations _____

   g. Self-help devices _____

   h. Surgical intervention _____

Copyright © 2019, Elsevier Inc. All Rights Reserved.

10. Identify general teaching methods for a(n):
    a. Infant
    b. Toddler
    c. Preschooler
    d. School-age child
    e. Older adult

11. A learner may find it difficult to concentrate in the presence of:

12. What characteristics does the patient need to learn psychomotor skills?

13. When selecting an environment for teaching, a nurse needs to consider:

14. Written materials used for teaching a patient with limited health literacy are usually presented at the

    _____ grade level.

15. Teaching sessions that are usually tolerated best last

    for _____ minutes. In planning the teaching session,

    essential information should be taught _____.

16. The patient becomes fatigued during the teaching session. You should:

17. For the nursing diagnosis *Lack of compliance with medication regimen related to insufficient knowledge of purpose and actions*, identify possible learning goals and outcomes and nursing interventions.

18. What is the preferred teaching style for the following types of learners?
    a. Visual
    b. Tactile
    c. Auditory

19. For the following, identify the domain of learning:
    a. Self-injection of insulin
    b. Coping with care of a family member
    c. Awareness of potential complications after a heart attack
    d. Response of the family to a member's substance abuse
    e. Sterile dressing technique
    f. Awareness of signs and symptoms of hypoglycemia

20. Identify an instructional technique that may be used in each of the following situations:
    a. A small group of patients in a cardiac rehabilitation group who need dietary information

    b. A patient with a leg cast who will be using crutches

    c. Students learning therapeutic communication skills to be used on a mental health unit

21. Explaining how a test will feel before the procedure is performed is an example of:

22. a. According to national reports, a total of _____ people in the United States have difficulty reading and understanding health information, including pamphlets and charts.
    b. What tools are available to assess your patients' literacy?

23. The nurse tells the patient that the injection will cause pain. What is a more effective way to communicate with the patient about the injection?

24. a. Identify what "teach-back" is and its purpose.

    b. Provide two examples of "teach-back" communication.

25. A focused assessment for patient education includes:

26. What should be included in the documentation of patient teaching?

27. Which of the following teaching strategies will promote patient participation? Select all that apply:

    a. Group discussion _____

    b. Question-and-answer sessions _____

    c. Lecture _____

    d. Role-play _____

    e. Simulation practice _____

Copyright © 2019, Elsevier Inc. All Rights Reserved.

28. Provide examples of how technology is used for teaching.

Select the best answer for each of the following questions:

29. A nurse is preparing to teach a group of new parents about infant care. The nurse recognizes that learning can be enhanced with:
    1. previous unfamiliarity with the topic area.
    2. fear of health outcomes.
    3. moderate discomfort.
    4. mild anxiety level.

30. The patient who most likely has the greatest motivation to learn is the individual who is:
    1. waiting for the results of diagnostic tests.
    2. hypertensive but has no symptoms.
    3. dealing with a family conflict.
    4. recovering from reconstructive surgery.

31. While preparing a teaching plan for a group of patients with diabetes, a nurse integrates the basic principle of education that:
    1. material should progress from complex to simpler ideas.
    2. prolonged teaching sessions improve concentration and attentiveness.
    3. learning is improved when more than one body sense is stimulated.
    4. previous knowledge of a topic area interferes with the acquisition of new information.

32. During a teaching session for a patient with heart disease, the nurse uses reinforcement to stimulate learning. An example of reinforcement for this patient is:
    1. allowing the patient to manage self-care needs.
    2. teaching about the disease process while delivering nursing care.
    3. outlining the exercise plan and providing explicit instructions.
    4. complimenting the patient on his or her ability to identify the action of prescribed medications.

33. After approximately 20 minutes have passed in the educational session, the nurse notices that the patient is slightly slumped in the chair and is no longer maintaining eye contact. The nurse should:
    1. reposition the patient in the chair.
    2. move the patient to a cooler, brighter room.
    3. reschedule the remainder of the teaching for another time.
    4. continue with the teaching session in order to cover the necessary content.

34. When preparing to teach the self-injection technique to a patient, the nurse begins with:
    1. having the patient demonstrate the procedure.
    2. discussing the procedure and the equipment used.
    3. providing written materials and having the patient practice the technique.
    4. demonstrating to the patient how to perform the procedure correctly.

35. After teaching a patient about a cerebrovascular accident (CVA/stroke), the nurse prepares to evaluate the patient's psychomotor domain of learning. This is accomplished by:
    1. observing the patient use a cane to ambulate.
    2. asking the patient about the basic etiology of a stroke.
    3. determining the patient's attitudes about the treatment regimen.
    4. having the patient complete a written schedule for daily activities at home.

36. When the teaching session has been completed, a nurse evaluates the patient's cognitive domain of learning to see if there are areas that require additional instruction. The nurse evaluates the patient's ability to:
    1. perform the range-of-motion exercises independently.
    2. identify the equipment necessary for surgical wound care.
    3. demonstrate the proper use of crutches to ambulate up and down stairs.
    4. discuss concerns about the difficulty in maintaining accurate records of the treatments.

37. Which patient appears to be demonstrating the greatest readiness to learn? The patient who says:
    1. "There's nothing wrong with me."
    2. "I think the doctor made a mistake."
    3. "I can manage on my own."
    4. "What do I need to know about this?"

38. A type of reinforcement that works well with children is:
    1. material.
    2. social.
    3. activity.
    4. negative.

39. A nurse recognizes that the most effective teaching strategy for a patient in the acceptance stage is to:
    1. share small bits of information.
    2. introduce only reality.
    3. provide simple explanations while doing care.
    4. focus on future skills and knowledge.

Copyright © 2019, Elsevier Inc. All Rights Reserved.

40. A patient is having difficulty communicating with other family members. Which one of the following would be the most effective teaching strategy for this patient?
    1. Demonstration
    2. Role-playing
    3. Telling
    4. Analogy

41. To teach a topic that is associated with coping with impaired function, the nurse will include information on:
    1. rehabilitation.
    2. laboratory tests.
    3. cause of the disease.
    4. screening measures.

42. Which of the following is an example of a correct teaching technique?
    1. Having a family member interpret information for the patient
    2. Using large-print materials for patients with decreased visual acuity
    3. Providing the same type of teaching plan for all patients with diabetes
    4. Teaching before the patient's bedtime

STUDY GROUP QUESTIONS

- What are the standards (e.g., The Joint Commission) for patient education?
- How does patient education promote, maintain, and restore health?
- What are the principles of teaching and learning?
- What factors may influence a patient's ability to learn?
- How does an individual's developmental status influence the selection of teaching methodologies?
- How does the teaching process compare with the communication and nursing processes?
- How does the nurse develop a teaching plan for a patient?
- What teaching approaches and instructional methods may be used by a nurse?
- How is patient education documented?

STUDY CHART

Develop sample teaching plans for patients who need to learn the following:
- Insulin injections
- 2-gm sodium diet

Continue building on the plans as you obtain further clinical practice and education.

Copyright © 2019, Elsevier Inc. All Rights Reserved.

13 Managing Patient Care

PRELIMINARY READING

Chapter 13, pp. 221–234

CASE STUDIES

1. As a nurse working on a busy surgical unit, this evening you have eight postoperative patients assigned to you.
   a. What types of activities could be delegated to an unlicensed nursing assistant?
   b. What determination do you need to make before safely delegating activities to the nursing assistant?
   c. What opportunities are available for doing more than one intervention at a time with the patient?

2. For these three patients in your assignment this evening, who will you see first and why?
   Patient #1, who has had prior respiratory difficulty, is currently using oxygen and watching TV. Evening meds are due to be given in 1 hour.
   Patient #2 is anxious and asking a lot of questions about the next day's surgery.
   Patient #3 had abdominal surgery this afternoon and has an intact and dry dressing and stable vital signs.

CHAPTER REVIEW

Match the description/definition in Column A with the correct term in Column B.

Column A	Column B
_____ 1. Responsibility	a. Allows decisions to be made at the staff level; shared governance is the typical structure used within health care organizations today
_____ 2. Autonomy	b. Contains the elements of respect and dignity, information sharing, participation, and collaboration
_____ 3. Transformational leadership	c. Individual responsibility for one's own actions
_____ 4. Delegation	d. Members of the group collaborate together to provide care as planned by the leader
_____ 5. Decentralized management	e. Freedom of choice and responsibility for those choices; ability to make independent decisions about the work of your unit such as scheduling or unit governance
_____ 6. Patient- and family-centered care model	f. One RN assumes the responsibility for a caseload of patients; the same nurse provides care for the same patients during their stay in a health care facility
_____ 7. Team nursing	g. Creating work environments that allow individuals to work to their highest potential and bring positive change to the work environment through their use of reflection, intellectual stimulation, and using the best evidence to guide their decisions
_____ 8. Authority	h. The process of assigning part of one person's responsibility to another qualified person in a specific situation
_____ 9. Accountability	i. The duties or tasks that you are required or expected to do
_____ 10. Primary nursing	j. The official power to act. It provides a nurse power to make final decisions and give instructions related to the decisions

Copyright © 2019, Elsevier Inc. All Rights Reserved.

Complete the following:

11. Identify three responsibilities of a nurse manager.

12. To implement transformational leadership, the nurse will use the TEEAMS approach. Identify the components of this approach:

    T -

    E -

    E -

    A -

    M -

    S -

13. The five rights of delegation are:

14. Identify an advantage and disadvantage of the total patient care model.

15. Case management is:

16. Provide at least one example of how staff members can be actively involved when decentralized decision-making exists on a nursing unit:

17. For the QSEN competency of Teamwork and Collaboration, identify ways that team communication can be promoted.

18. A patient on the unit, who was admitted 2 days ago with ketoacidosis, has a blood glucose level of 425, which is far above the expected range. The patient was receiving a longer-acting insulin. There are concerns about the type of insulin and dietary management. Identify the way this information should be reported with the SBAR:

    S -

    B -

    A -

    R -

Select the best answer for each of the following questions:

19. A student nurse is working with a patient who has begun to have respiratory difficulty. It is the student nurse's initial responsibility to:
    1. call the pharmacy.
    2. alert the primary nurse.
    3. contact the attending physician.
    4. administer the prescribed medication.

20. The nurses on a medical unit are discussing plans to change the focus of the unit to the primary nursing care model. With this model, the assignment for nurse A is:
    1. Mrs. J., Mrs. R., and Mrs. T. for the length of their stays.
    2. to receive reports from the nursing assistant on the care of Mrs. J., Mrs. R., and Mrs. T.
    3. side 1 of the unit in cooperation with nurse B and the nursing assistant.
    4. medication administration for all of the patients on the unit while nurse B does the physical care with the nursing assistant.

21. A nurse in the long-term care facility is delegating care to the nursing assistant. It is appropriate for the nurse to delegate the care of the patient who requires:
    1. hygienic care.
    2. an admission history.
    3. administration of oral medications.
    4. vital sign measurements after episodes of arrhythmias.

22. A student nurse is assigned to care for a patient in the hospital. The student is unable to obtain the patient's blood pressure reading after two attempts. The student should:
    1. keep trying to get the blood pressure measurement.
    2. use the closest measurement to the last reading.
    3. ask another nurse to obtain the blood pressure measurement.
    4. inform the instructor about the difficulty and request assistance.

23. A nurse is working with a patient who has just returned from surgery. The nurse has no experience working with the patient's postoperative surgical dressing. During an assessment, the nurse notices that the dressing has come loose and has fallen away from the surgical wound. The patient tells the nurse, "Oh, you can fix it." The nurse:
    1. asks the patient to help replace the dressing.
    2. replaces the loosened dressing as best as possible.
    3. asks the surgeon to replace the dressing.
    4. covers the wound with a sterile dry dressing until assistance is obtained.

45

Copyright © 2019, Elsevier Inc. All Rights Reserved.

24. A nurse has been assigned to work on a very busy medical unit in the hospital. It is important for the nurse to employ time management skills. The nurse implements a plan to:
    1. have all the patients' major needs met in the early morning hours.
    2. anticipate possible interruptions by therapists and visitors.
    3. complete assessments and treatments for each patient at different times each day.
    4. leave each day unstructured to allow for changes in treatments and patient assignments.

25. The staff on a medical unit in an acute care facility is moving to a system where the nurse manager will lead a group of other RNs, LPNs, and aides. This is an example of:
    1. functional nursing.
    2. primary nursing.
    3. total patient care.
    4. team nursing.

26. A student nurse has a multiple patient assignment. In reviewing the report obtained from the primary nurse, the student should decide to see which patient first? The patient who is:
    1. experiencing nausea.
    2. using a bedpan.
    3. having an episode of severe dyspnea.
    4. thirsty and wants another drink with breakfast.

27. A nursing manager supports staff involvement through a variety of ways. The new nurse is seeking to learn these positive strategies but would question:
    1. the establishment of nursing practice committees.
    2. restriction of staff input for patient assignments.
    3. promotion of interprofessional collaboration.
    4. arrangement of staff rounds for health care professionals from different disciplines.

STUDY GROUP QUESTIONS

- To whom may a nurse delegate care responsibilities? What types of responsibilities may be delegated legally and safely?
- What is involved in decentralized decision making?
- How does the nurse manager function within the health care team?
- How do the different types of nursing care delivery models differ from one another?
- How does interprofessional collaboration improve the quality of patient care?
- What is necessary for effective coordination and prioritization of care?

STUDY CHART

Create a study chart to compare and contrast the different *Nursing Care Delivery Models*.

Copyright © 2019, Elsevier Inc. All Rights Reserved.

14 Infection Prevention and Control

PRELIMINARY READING

Chapter 14, pp. 235–267

CASE STUDIES

1. An 86-year-old woman in an extended care facility has a urinary catheter attached to a drainage system.
   a. What precautions should be taken for this patient to prevent a urinary tract infection?

2. Yesterday a 45-year-old man had abdominal surgery. He has a large midline abdominal incision covered by a sterile dressing. He will require dressing changes twice daily.
   a. What precautions should be taken for this patient to prevent wound infection?

3. An 85-year-old man with MRSA requires isolation precautions. He is oriented to his surroundings and is concerned about whether his family will be able to visit him.
   a. What specific nursing care should be implemented for this patient?

CHAPTER REVIEW

Match the description/definition in Column A with the correct term in Column B.

Column A	Column B
_____ 1. Arises from microorganisms outside the patient	a. Inflammatory exudate
_____ 2. Cellular response to injury or infection	b. Aseptic technique
_____ 3. Microorganisms that cause another infection because they are resistant to antibiotics	c. Health care–acquired infection
_____ 4. Infection that developed that was not present at the time of patient admission	d. Sterilization
_____ 5. Methods to reduce or eliminate disease-producing micro-organisms	e. Colonization
_____ 6. Microorganisms that do not cause disease but help to maintain health	f. Inflammation
_____ 7. Process that eliminates all forms of microbial life	g. Flora
_____ 8. Disease-producing microorganism	h. Pathogen
_____ 9. Fluid, dead cells, and WBCs that drain from an affected site	i. Endogenous infection
_____ 10. Microorganism that grows but does not cause disease	j. Suprainfection
_____ 11. Ability of microorganisms to produce disease	k. Exogenous infection
_____ 12. Being more than normally vulnerable to a disease	l. Virulence
_____ 13. Alteration of a patient's flora with a resulting overgrowth	m. Susceptibility

47

Copyright © 2019, Elsevier Inc. All Rights Reserved.

Complete the following:

14. Identify whether the following are performed using sterile technique in an acute care environment:

    a. Hand hygiene _____

    b. Postoperative dressing change _____

    c. Urinary catheter insertion _____

    d. Barrier precautions _____

    e. Intramuscular injection _____

15. An outcome for a patient with a 3-cm-diameter wound is:

16. Immunizations are available for which of the following? Select all that apply.

    a. Hepatitis A _____

    b. Diphtheria _____

    c. Rubella _____

    d. Tuberculosis _____

    e. AIDS _____

    f. Varicella _____

17. For the following, select all actions that require that equipment be discarded and/or the sterile field be re-done.

    a. A mask is worn when opening the sterile tray. _____

    b. The sterile dressing package is torn. _____

    c. The tip of the sterile syringe touches the surface of a clean, disposable glove. _____

    d. A sterile basin is held out over the sterile field. _____

    e. A cup on the sterile field is touched with a sterile gloved hand. _____

    f. Sterile dressings are placed within the 1-inch edge of the sterile field. _____

18. Identify specific actions that a nurse can implement to interrupt the chain of infection.

    a. Control or eliminate the infectious agent:

    b. Control or eliminate the reservoir:

    c. Control the portals of exit:

    d. Control transmission:

    e. Control susceptibility of host:

19. What results would be expected for the following laboratory studies in the presence of an infection?

    a. WBC count

    b. Erythrocyte sedimentation rate

    c. Iron level

    d. Neutrophils

    e. Basophils

20. In relation to health care–acquired infections (HAI):

    a. How can they be reduced?

    b. Which patients are more susceptible?

21. A patient's gastrointestinal defenses against infection are altered by:

22. Select all the appropriate techniques for isolation precautions.

    a. Wash hands in the clean utility room after patient care. _____

    b. Provide for the patient's sensory needs during care. _____

    c. Prevent visitors from entering the patient's room. _____

    d. Keep face mask below the level of eyeglasses or goggles. _____

    e. Place disposable items in paper bags. _____

    f. Keep PPE at the door to the room or in an anteroom area. _____

23. Handling of biohazardous waste includes:

24. Specify the order in which the following PPE should be applied before entering an isolation room:

    a. Mask _____

    b. Gloves _____

    c. Gown _____

Copyright © 2019, Elsevier Inc. All Rights Reserved.

25. If a mask, gown, and gloves are worn into an isolation room, the first item of PPE that is removed when exiting the room is/are the:

26. Select all of the following in which appropriate asepsis has occurred:

    a. Handling a sterile dressing with clean gloves _____

    b. Holding a sterile bowl above waist level using sterile gloves _____

    c. Keeping the hands above the elbows after a surgical scrub _____

    d. Turning away from and placing one's back to the sterile field _____

    e. Talking or coughing over the sterile field _____

    f. Discarding sterile packages that are wet _____

    g. Placing objects to the edge of the sterile field _____

    h. Discarding a small amount of solution before pouring the remainder into a sterile container on the field _____

27. For the nursing diagnosis *altered skin integrity, related to 2-inch-diameter pressure ulcer on sacrum*, identify a patient outcome and nursing interventions.

28. Number the flaps on the sterile package in the figure according to which should be opened first, second, and last.

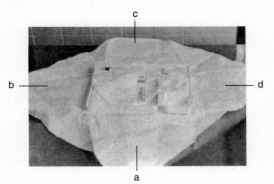

29. Proper disposal of contaminated sharps includes:

30. Provide an example of how the nurse needs to be aware of his or her own breaks in aseptic technique.

31. What equipment is needed to collect a urine specimen from the patient with an indwelling urinary catheter?

32. Select all of the following actions that are appropriate for hand washing with antimicrobial soap and water.

    a. Cleaning under fingernails _____

    b. Removing rings during washing _____

    c. Leaning against the sink _____

    d. Keeping the water temperature hot _____

    e. Washing the hands for at least 15 seconds _____

    f. Turning off the faucet with the elbows _____

    g. Keeping hands and forearms lower than the elbows during washing _____

    h. Drying from the elbows to the fingers _____

33. The patient sees the nurse using the hand sanitizer frequently and remarks, "I must be full of germs since you're always cleaning your hands." How should the nurse respond?

34. Information on the current immunizations schedule can be found at the:

35. One of the most common infections in long-term care (LTC) is:

36. Which of the following infectious organisms are transmitted through blood? Select all that apply.

    a. *Candida albicans* (fungi) _____

    b. HIV _____

    c. *Staphlococcus aureus* _____

    d. *Plasmodium falciparum* (protozoa) _____

    e. streptococcus _____

    f. hepatitis B _____

Copyright © 2019, Elsevier Inc. All Rights Reserved.

37. Place the following steps for specimen collection in an isolation room in the correct order. After changing the bed linens, the gloves have been changed, then the nurse should:

a. Perform hand hygiene _____

b. Check the container label and send the specimen to the lab _____

c. Place the specimen container on a clean paper towel in the bathroom _____

d. Transfer the specimen to the containers _____

e. Collect the specimen _____

38. When splashing or spraying of bodily fluids is anticipated, the nurse should use a:

39. Identify the breaks in isolation technique in the photos below:

40. Indicate the type of immunity for each of the following:

a. Having measles as a child _____

b. A baby receiving its mother's antibodies _____

c. Being immunized for influenza _____

41. Identify how the following factors influence an individual's susceptibility to infection:
a. Heredity

b. Inadequate defenses

c. Environment

42. Which of the following items are considered *noncritical* and must be cleaned but not usually sterilized? Select all that apply.

a. Bedpans _____

b. Endoscopes _____

c. Linens _____

d. Blood pressure cuffs _____

e. Surgical instruments _____

f. Stethoscopes _____

43. What do you do if your gloves are torn and your hands come in contact with a contaminated article or body fluids?

44. a. Identify two multidrug-resistant organisms (MDROs).

b. Which MDRO is hardest to eliminate and why?

45. An alcohol-based hand sanitizer is the preferred method for cleaning the hands when working in a healthcare facility when the hands are not visibly dirty.

True _____   False _____

Copyright © 2019, Elsevier Inc. All Rights Reserved.

46. Put the following steps for sterile gloving in order:
   a. With thumb and first two fingers of nondominant hand, grasp glove for dominant hand by touching only inside surface of cuff. _____

   b. Grasp inner package and lay on clean, dry, flat surface at waist level. Open package, keeping gloves on inside surface of wrapper. _____

   c. With gloved dominant hand, slip fingers underneath cuff of second glove. Carefully pull second glove over fingers of nondominant hand. _____

   d. Identify right and left glove. Each glove has a cuff approximately 5 cm (2 inches) wide. Glove dominant hand first. _____

   e. Remove outer glove package wrapper by carefully separating and peeling apart sides. _____

   f. Carefully pull glove over dominant hand, leaving a cuff and being sure that cuff does not roll up wrist. Be sure that thumb and fingers are in proper spaces. _____

Select the best answer for each of the following questions:

47. At the community health fair, a nurse is asked by one of the residents about the influenza vaccine. The nurse responds to the resident that the influenza vaccine is strongly recommended for individuals who are:
   1. health care workers.
   2. traveling to other countries.
   3. younger than 6 years of age.
   4. between 40 and 65 years of age.

48. A nurse is preparing a room for a patient with tuberculosis. The specific aspect for this tier of Standard Precautions that is different than tier 1 is that the care should include:
   1. a private room with negative air flow.
   2. hand hygiene after gloves are removed.
   3. eye protection if splashing is possible.
   4. disposal of sharps in a puncture-resistant container.

49. A nurse is preparing a teaching plan for patients about the hepatitis B virus. The nurse informs them that this virus may be transmitted by:
   1. mosquitoes.
   2. droplet nuclei.
   3. blood products.
   4. improperly handled food.

50. A nurse is working on a unit with a number of patients who have infectious diseases. One of the most important methods for reducing the spread of microorganisms is:
   1. sterilization of equipment.
   2. the use of gloves and gowns.
   3. maintenance of isolation precautions.
   4. hand hygiene before and after patient care.

51. The assignment today for a nurse includes a patient with tuberculosis. In caring for a patient on droplet precautions, the nurse should routinely use:
   1. regular masks and eyewear.
   2. regular gowns and gloves.
   3. surgical hand hygiene and gloves.
   4. particulate filtration masks and gowns.

52. A nurse is caring for a patient who has a large abdominal wound that requires a sterile saline soak and dressing. While performing the care, the nurse drops the saline-soaked 4 × 4 gauze near the wound on the patient's abdomen. The nurse should:
   1. discontinue the procedure.
   2. throw the gauze away and prepare a new 4 × 4 gauze.
   3. pick up the 4 × 4 with sterile forceps and place it on the wound.
   4. rinse the 4 × 4 with saline and place it on the wound using sterile gloves.

53. A nurse is checking the laboratory results of a male patient admitted to the medical unit. The nurse is alerted to the presence of an infectious process based on the finding of:
   1. Iron: 80 g/100 mL.
   2. Neutrophils: 65%.
   3. Erythrocyte sedimentation rate (ESR): 13 mm per hour.
   4. White blood cells (WBC): 16,000/mm^3

54. The individual most at risk for a latex allergy is the patient with a history of:
   1. hypertension.
   2. congenital heart disease.
   3. diabetes mellitus.
   4. cholecystitis.

55. A nurse is working with a patient who has a deep laceration to the right lower extremity. To specifically reduce a possible reservoir of infection, the nurse:
   1. wears gloves and a mask at all times.
   2. isolates the patient's personal articles.
   3. has the patient cover the mouth and nose when coughing.
   4. changes the dressing to the extremity when it becomes soiled.

Copyright © 2019, Elsevier Inc. All Rights Reserved.

56. A nurse implements droplet precautions (smaller than 5 microns) for the patient with:
    1. pulmonary tuberculosis.
    2. varicella.
    3. rubella.
    4. herpes.

57. A patient who has had a transplant will require what type of isolation?
    1. Contact
    2. Airborne
    3. Droplet
    4. Protective

58. For a patient with hepatitis A, the nurse is aware that the disease is transmitted through:
    1. feces.
    2. blood.
    3. skin.
    4. droplet nuclei.

59. A sign that is indicative of a systemic infection resulting from a wound is:
    1. redness.
    2. drainage.
    3. edema.
    4. fever.

60. There are small open wounds on the hands of the nurse. The nurse's most appropriate action is:
    1. asking to work at the nurse's station for the day.
    2. using clean, disposable gloves for patient care.
    3. applying antibacterial ointment before patient contact.
    4. providing patient care as usual and washing the hands more frequently.

61. A nurse is aware that older adults are more susceptible to infection as a result of:
    1. thickening of the dermal and epidermal skin layers.
    2. increased production of T lymphocytes.
    3. increased production of digestive juices.
    4. drying of the oral mucosa.

62. The Zika virus is an example of which type of transmission route?
    1. Water
    2. Food
    3. Feces
    4. Vector

63. Which of the following places the patient at a greater risk for infection?
    1. Allowing backflow from the urine drainage bag to the bladder
    2. Providing frequent oral hygiene
    3. Covering draining wounds
    4. Keeping patients from lying on tubes

STUDY GROUP QUESTIONS

- What is the nature of the infectious process?
- What are the components of the chain of infection?
- What are the body's normal defenses against infection?
- What is a health care–associated infection, who are the patients at greatest risk, and how can a nurse prevent this type of infection?
- How is the nursing process applied to infection control in the acute, extended care, and home care environments?
- What nursing measures may be implemented to prevent or control the spread of infection?
- What is included in Standard Precautions (Tier 1)?
- What are the different types of transmission-based (Tier 2) precautions?
- What information may be taught to the patient and the patient's family for prevention or control of infectious processes?
- How does the nurse perform the procedures that are important for infection control, including hand hygiene, sterile gloving, application of PPE, and specimen collection?

STUDY CHART

Create a study chart to compare the different types of isolation and safety precautions for patients.

Copyright © 2019, Elsevier Inc. All Rights Reserved.

15 Vital Signs

PRELIMINARY READING

Chapter 15, pp. 268–317

CASE STUDIES

1. You are volunteering at a community health fair. You have been asked to take blood pressure (BP) readings for the residents participating in the event.
   a. What blood pressure readings indicate that follow-up care should be recommended?
   b. What other information may be obtained from a patient while taking the blood pressure reading?

2. You are assigned to an orthopedic unit in the medical center. A patient was involved in an automobile accident and has bilateral casts on the upper arms.
   a. How will you obtain the patient's pulse rate and blood pressure?

3. You have just started your shift at the extended care facility. The nurse going off duty reports that one of your assigned patents is febrile.
   a. What signs and symptoms do you expect to find with a patient who is febrile?
   b. What interventions are indicated for febrile patients?

4. The patient has been brought to the emergency room with signs of heat stroke.
   a. What interventions are anticipated for this patient?
   b. What teaching should be done to prevent the occurrence in the future?

5. A postoperative patient is being monitored with pulse oximetry. You are checking the reading, but the device does not appear to be working.
   a. What are the expected readings for oxygen saturation?
   b. What "troubleshooting" can you perform to determine if the pulse oximeter is working properly?
   c. How can you help the postoperative patient to improve his or her saturation level?

6. You are examining a laceration on the patient's left lower leg. The patient tells you that she got the wound over two weeks ago and it doesn't appear to be healing. Diabetes mellitus has been ruled out, so you are looking for signs of peripheral vascular disease.
   a. What signs are indicative of altered arterial circulation to the lower extremities?
   b. If peripheral vascular disease is present, what do you expect to find when you measure pulses?

Copyright © 2019, Elsevier Inc. All Rights Reserved.

CHAPTER REVIEW

Match the description/definition in Column A with the correct term in Column B.

Column A

_____ 1. Decrease of systolic and diastolic pressures below normal

_____ 2. Another word for fever

_____ 3. Difference between the apical and radial pulse rates

_____ 4. Widening of blood vessels

_____ 5. Pulse rate less than 60 beats per minute for an adult

_____ 6. Above 140/90 mm Hg for two or more readings

_____ 7. Rate of breathing abnormally rapid

_____ 8. Decreased body temperature

_____ 9. No respirations for several seconds

_____ 10. Rate of breathing abnormally slow

_____ 11. Normal breathing

_____ 12. Temporary disappearance of sounds between Korotkoff sounds

Column B

a. Tachypnea

b. Bradypnea

c. Hypothermia

d. Apnea

e. Bradycardia

f. Hypotension

g. Pulse deficit

h. Hypertension

i. Vasodilation

j. Febrile

k. Auscultatory gap

l. Eupnea

Complete the following:

13. Convert the following temperature readings:

 a. 97°F = _____°C

 b. 38.4°C = _____°F

 c. 102°F = _____°C

 d. 39.4°C = _____°F

14. What are the Fahrenheit and centigrade temperature readings that should alert the nurse to an alteration in the patient's temperature regulation?

15. Indicate on the model where the following pulses should be palpated:
 a. Carotid
 b. Brachial
 c. Radial
 d. Apical
 e. Dorsalis pedis

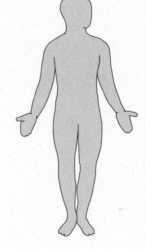

16. Indicate on the aneroid scale where the following blood pressure reading would be noted:
 Korotkoff sounds first heard at 164 mm Hg and inaudible at 92 mm Hg

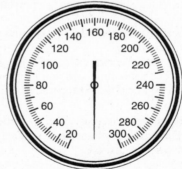

17. Apical pulse measurements may not be delegated to unlicensed assistive personnel.

 True _____ False _____

18. Identify actions that will reduce body temperature in the following ways:
 a. Conduction:
 b. Convection:
 c. Evaporation:

19. A patient is on isolation precautions, and temperature measurements are being used to monitor the status of the fever. The thermometer of choice in this situation is a(n):

54

Chapter **15** Vital Signs

Copyright © 2019, Elsevier Inc. All Rights Reserved.

20. A nurse identifies a pulse deficit. How was this assessed?

21. For a patient who has had a right mastectomy, the nurse should take the blood pressure:

22. Vital signs are usually recorded on the:

23. Decreasing hemoglobin levels will _____ the respiratory rate.

24. To obtain arterial oxygen saturation for an adult patient, the pulse oximeter may be applied to:

25. The pulse pressure for a patient with a BP of 150/90 is:

26. Which of the following are correct for blood pressure measurement? Select all that apply.

   a. The cuff is 40% of the circumference of the limb being used. _____

   b. The bladder encircles 50% of the arm of an adult. _____

   c. The cuff is deflated at a rate of 2 to 3 mm Hg per second. _____

   d. The arm is kept below the level of the heart. _____

   e. The cuff is inflated to 30 mm Hg above the point where the pulse disappears. _____

   f. The systolic blood pressure is identified as the first onset of Korotkoff sounds. _____

   g. A difference of 30 mm Hg is expected between the left and right arm measurements. _____

27. A nurse is preparing to take the patient's oral temperature, but discovers that he has just had a cup of coffee. The appropriate action is to:

28. Identify a situation when a patient's blood pressure may need to be palpated.

29. How are the following vital signs measured differently in children than in adults?
   a. Temperature:
   b. Blood pressure:

30. Which of the following are correct techniques for a tympanic temperature measurement? Select all that apply:

   a. Using the right ear if the patient has been lying on his/her left side in bed. _____

   b. Pointing the probe midpoint between the eyebrows and sideburns for children younger than 3 years of age. _____

   c. Pulling the ear pinna backward and down for an adult. _____

   d. Moving the thermometer back and forth a little during the assessment. _____

   e. Fitting the speculum tip loosely into the ear canal _____

   f. Waiting 2 to 3 minutes before repeating the measurement in the same ear. _____

31. A patient's pulse is expected to be increased in the presence of which of the following factors? Select all that apply.

   a. Anxiety _____

   b. Hypothermia _____

   c. Unrelieved severe pain _____

   d. Presence of asthma _____

   e. Hemorrhage _____

   f. Administration of beta blockers _____

32. What are the contraindications for the following temperature assessments?
   a. Axillary temperature
   b. Rectal temperature

33. End-tidal carbon dioxide ($ETCO_2$) values are used commonly for patients with:

55

Copyright © 2019, Elsevier Inc. All Rights Reserved.

34. For a blood pressure taken in the lower extremity:
    a. How should the patient be positioned?
    b. What artery is used for palpation?
    c. Is the reading expected to be higher or lower than in the upper extremity?

35. Place the following steps for apical pulse measurement in the correct order:

    a. Count the rate for one minute. _____

    b. Replace the gown and position the patient for comfort. _____

    c. Locate anatomical landmarks. _____

    d. Place the diaphragm over the 5th intercostal space at the left midclavicular line. _____

    e. Warm the diaphragm in the hand for 5–10 seconds. _____

    f. Position the patient supine or sitting. _____

36. The danger of an increased temperature in young children is the potential for:

37. a. Provide three examples of antipyretic medications that may be ordered for a febrile patient.

    b. After administration of an antipyretic, when should the temperature be taken?

38. For orthostatic hypotension:
    a. How is it assessed?

    b. What are some of the factors that place an individual at risk?

39. Indicate the following for core temperature readings:
    a. Readings are invasive or noninvasive?
    b. Sites for core readings include:

40. What are the uses for the diaphragm and the bell of the stethoscope?

41. Indicate whether the body temperature is increased or decreased for the following individuals:
    a. Ovulating female
    b. Older adult
    c. An individual who has exercised
    d. A patient in the OR having surgery
    e. An individual under stress
    f. A well person at 6:30 A.M.

42. Indicate the correct techniques for pulse oximetry. Select all that apply.
    a. Recording the first reading after application of the probe. _____

    b. Using the earlobe for a patient with tremors. _____

    c. Applying the probe to the bridge of a toddler's nose. _____

    d. Using fingers with acrylic nails, but no nail polish. _____

    e. Expecting readings between 80% and 90%. _____

    f. Changing the site of a continuous monitor every 2 hours. _____

43. How do the following influence respiration?
    a. Anxiety:
    b. Analgesic medications:
    c. Body position:
    d. Abdominal incision:
    e. Exercise:

44. Which of the following can lead to hypotension? Select all that apply.

    a. Hemorrhage. _____

    b. Stress. _____

    c. Obesity. _____

    d. Fluid deficit. _____

    e. Cigarette smoking. _____

45. The peripheral pulse is irregular. What should the nurse do?

Copyright © 2019, Elsevier Inc. All Rights Reserved.

46. Which of the following will lead to false-high blood pressure readings? Select all that apply.

   a. Bladder or cuff too narrow or too short _____

   b. Cuff wrapped too loosely or unevenly _____

   c. Deflating cuff too quickly _____

   d. Arm below heart level _____

   e. Repeating assessments too quickly _____

   f. Inadequate inflation level _____

47. Respirations are affected by the patient's oxygen carrying capacity in the blood. Identify the expected values for the complete blood count (CBC).
   a. Hemoglobin
   b. Hematocrit
   c. Red blood cell count

48. The patient is hypothermic. Which of the following actions are appropriate? Select all that apply:

   a. Apply warm blankets. _____

   b. Offer warm liquids. _____

   c. Reduce external body coverings. _____

   d. Administer antipyretic, if ordered. _____

   e. Remove wet clothing or linen. _____

   f. Limit physical activity. _____

49. Factors that contribute to hypertension include:

50. The patient's condition has worsened over the last few hours. What should be done for the patient's vital signs?

51. What is the correct procedure for taking a temporal artery temperature?

Select the best answer for each of the following questions:

52. A nurse is working on a pediatric unit and assessing the vital signs of an infant admitted for gastroenteritis. The nurse expects that the vital signs are normally the following (BP is blood pressure in units of mm Hg, P is pulse rate in units of beats per minute, and R is respirations in units of breaths per minute):
   1. BP = 90/50, P = 122, R = 46.
   2. BP = 90/60, P = 80, R = 20.
   3. BP = 100/60, P = 140, R = 32.
   4. BP = 110/50, P = 98, R = 40.

53. While working in an extended care facility, a nurse expects the vital signs of an older adult patient to be:
   1. BP = 98/70, P = 60, R = 12.
   2. BP = 120/60, P = 110, R = 30.
   3. BP = 140/90, P = 74, R = 14.
   4. BP = 150/100, P = 90, R = 25.

54. A student nurse is taking vital signs for her assigned patients on the surgical unit. The student is aware that a patient's body temperature may be reduced after:
   1. exercise.
   2. emotional stress.
   3. periods of sleep.
   4. cigarette smoking.

55. While working in an emergency department, a nurse is carefully monitoring the vital signs of the patients who have been admitted. The nurse is alert to the potential for a decrease in a patient's pulse rate as a result of:
   1. hemorrhage.
   2. hypothyroidism.
   3. respiratory difficulty.
   4. epinephrine (adrenaline) administration.

56. A patient is being treated for hyperthermia. The nurse anticipates that the patient's response to this condition will be:
   1. generalized pallor.
   2. bradycardia.
   3. reduced thirst.
   4. diaphoresis.

57. Several friends have gone on a ski trip and have been exposed to very cold temperatures. One of the individuals appears to be slightly hypothermic. The best initial response by the nurse in the ski lodge is to give this individual:
   1. soup.
   2. coffee.
   3. brandy.
   4. warm cola.

58. When checking the temperature of a patient, a nurse notes that he is febrile. A nonsteroidal antipyretic medication is ordered. The nurse prepares to administer:
   1. digoxin.
   2. prednisone.
   3. theophylline.
   4. acetaminophen.

59. A nurse has been assigned a number of different patients in the long-term care unit. When taking vital signs, the nurse is alert to the greater possibility of tachycardia for the patient with:
   1. anemia.
   2. hypothyroidism.
   3. a temperature of 98°F.
   4. a patient-controlled analgesic (PCA) pump with morphine drip.

57

Copyright © 2019, Elsevier Inc. All Rights Reserved.

60. While reviewing the vital signs taken by the aide this morning, a nurse notes that one of the patients is hypotensive. The nurse will be checking to see if the patient is experiencing:
    1. lightheadedness.
    2. a decreased heart rate.
    3. an increased urinary output.
    4. increased warmth to the skin.

61. Vital sign measurements have been completed on all assigned patients. The nurse will need to immediately report a finding of:
    1. pulse pressure of 40 mm Hg.
    2. apical pulses of 78, 80, 76 beats per minute.
    3. apical pulse of 82 beats per minute; radial pulse of 70 beats per minute.
    4. BP of 140/80 mm Hg left arm, 136/74 mm Hg right arm.

62. A nurse is preparing to take vital signs for the patients on the acute care unit. A tympanic temperature assessment is indicated for the patient:
    1. after rectal surgery.
    2. wearing a hearing aid.
    3. experiencing otitis media.
    4. after an exercise session.

63. Which of the following is a correct technique for blood pressure monitoring?
    1. Placing the cuff over rolled up or thick clothing
    2. Putting the cuff firmly on the antecubital space
    3. Inflating the cuff to 60 mm Hg above patient's usual systolic pressure
    4. Having the patient rest for 5 minutes before measurement

64. A 34-year-old patient has gone to a physician's office for an annual physical examination. The nurse is completing the vital signs before the patient is seen by the physician. The nurse alerts the physician to a finding of:
    1. T: 37.6° C.
    2. P: 120 beats per minute.
    3. R: 18 breaths per minute.
    4. BP: 116/78 mm Hg.

65. A nurse is assigned to the well-child center that is affiliated with the acute care facility. A mother takes her $1\frac{1}{2}$-year-old son to the center for his immunizations. The nurse assesses the child's pulse rate by checking the:
    1. radial artery.
    2. apical artery.
    3. popliteal artery.
    4. femoral artery.

66. A nurse determines that a patient's pulse rate is significantly lower than it has been during the past week. The nurse reassesses and finds that the pulse rate is still 46 beats per minute. The nurse should first:
    1. document the measurement.
    2. administer a stimulant medication.
    3. inform the charge nurse or physician.
    4. apply 100% oxygen at maximum flow rate.

67. The most important sign of heat stroke is:
    1. hot, dry skin.
    2. nausea.
    3. excessive thirst.
    4. muscle cramping.

68. The most accurate temperature measurement for an adult patient experiencing tachypnea and dyspnea is:
    1. oral.
    2. forehead.
    3. axillary.
    4. tympanic.

69. A nurse should insert a rectal thermometer into the adult patient:
    1. $\frac{1}{4}$ to $\frac{1}{2}$ inch.
    2. 1 to $1\frac{1}{2}$ inches.
    3. $1\frac{1}{2}$ to 2 inches.
    4. 2 to $2\frac{1}{2}$ inches.

70. An adolescent patient is expected to have a respiratory rate that is:
    1. 35–40/minute.
    2. 30–50/minute.
    3. 25–32/minute.
    4. 16–20/minute.

71. Which of the following values indicates the correct pulse pressure for a patient with a blood pressure of 170/90?
    1. 80
    2. 170
    3. 260
    4. Value not known based on the information given

72. For a patient who is experiencing a febrile state, the nurse should:
    1. ambulate the patient frequently.
    2. restrict fluid intake.
    3. keep the patient warm.
    4. provide oxygen as ordered.

73. A nurse anticipates that bradycardia will be evident if a patient is:
    1. exercising.
    2. hypothermic.
    3. asthmatic.
    4. extremely anxious.

   Copyright © 2019, Elsevier Inc. All Rights Reserved.

74. A nurse anticipates that a patient with hypertension will be receiving:
    1. diuretics.
    2. antipyretics.
    3. narcotic analgesics.
    4. anticholinergics.

75. To determine the arterial blood flow to a patient's feet, the nurse should assess the:
    1. radial artery.
    2. brachial artery.
    3. popliteal artery.
    4. dorsalis pedis artery.

76. A nurse anticipates an increase in blood pressure for the patient who is:
    1. sleeping.
    2. overweight.
    3. taking narcotics.
    4. hemorrhaging.

77. Prehypertension is classified as an average of repeated readings of:
    1. Systolic: 120 to 139 mm Hg; diastolic: 80 to 89 mm Hg.
    2. Systolic: 140 to 159 mm Hg; diastolic: 90 to 99 mm Hg.
    3. Systolic: 160 to 179 mm Hg; diastolic: 90 to 99 mm Hg.
    4. Systolic: greater than 180 mm Hg: diastolic; greater than 100 mm Hg.

78. Which sign or symptom is indicative of high blood pressure?
    1. Dizziness
    2. Headache
    3. Restlessness
    4. Cool skin over the extremities

79. The patient has a fever that spikes and then shows acceptable temperature levels. The temperature returns to acceptable two to three times within a 24-hour period. This is documented by the nurse as:
    1. sustained.
    2. remittent.
    3. relapsing.
    4. intermittent.

80. An electronic blood pressure measurement is acceptable for a patient who:
    1. is shivering.
    2. has had fluctuations in readings.
    3. requires frequent monitoring.
    4. has an irregular heart beat.

81. Which of the following observations of the newly hired nurse requires intervention by the nurse manager?
    1. Fabric covering the stethoscope
    2. Use of 12" long tubing
    3. Use of the bell to auscultate heart sounds
    4. Cleansing the stethoscope with alcohol in between patients

82. The nurse assesses the patient's pulse as diminished and barely palpable. This is documented as
    1. +1.
    2. +2.
    3. +3.
    4. +4.

83. The nurse in the Emergency Department assesses that the patient's respirations are below the expected amount. The nurse recognizes that slow respirations can be indicative of:
    1. pneumonia.
    2. hemorrhage.
    3. hypoglycemia.
    4. brain stem trauma.

STUDY GROUP QUESTIONS

- What are the guidelines for measurement of vital signs?
- When should vital signs be taken?
- How does the nurse determine what sites and equipment to use for measurement of vital signs?
- What body processes regulate temperature?
- What factors influence body temperature?
- How is the temperature measurement converted from Centigrade to Fahrenheit and vice versa?
- What sites and equipment are used for temperature measurement?
- What nursing interventions are appropriate for increases and decreases in a patient's body temperature?
- What factors influence pulse rate?
- What sites may be used for pulse rate assessment?
- How should the stethoscope be used in pulse rate assessment?
- What changes may occur in the pulse rate and rhythm?
- What nursing interventions are appropriate for alterations in pulse rate?
- What is blood pressure?
- What factors may increase or decrease blood pressure?
- What are abnormal alterations in blood pressure?
- What equipment is used for blood pressure measurement?
- What nursing interventions are appropriate for increases and decreases in blood pressure?
- What body processes are involved in respiration?
- How are respirations assessed?
- What alterations may be noted in a patient's respirations?

Copyright © 2019, Elsevier Inc. All Rights Reserved.

- How does pulse oximetry function and what is its purpose?
- What are the procedures for assessment of temperature, pulse rate, respirations, blood pressure, and pulse oxygen saturation?
- What should be included in patient and family teaching for measurement and evaluation of vital signs?

Create a study chart to compare the *Vital Signs Across the Life Span* that identifies expected temperature, pulse rate, respiration, and blood pressure for each age group, as well as changes in measurement techniques for the different age groups.

Copyright © 2019, Elsevier Inc. All Rights Reserved.

16 Health Assessment and Physical Examination

PRELIMINARY READING

Chapter 16, pp. 318–378

CASE STUDIES

1. You are assigned to assist with physical examinations in the outpatient clinic. On the schedule for today are three patients. One of the patients is a 72-year-old Hispanic woman, another is a 16-year-old girl, and the last is a 4-year-old boy.
   a. How can you assist each of these patients to feel more at ease before and during the physical examination?

2. A patient in the physician's office informs you that he is having trouble hearing when other people are speaking to him.
   a. What specific assessments will you perform on this patient?

3. You observe a lesion on the patient's abdomen that is draining fluid.
   a. What specific assessments should be made?
   b. How should you prepare to assess the lesion?

CHAPTER REVIEW

Match the description/definition in Column A with the correct term in Column B.

	Column A	Column B
_____	1. Bluish discoloration of the lips, mouth, and conjunctivae	a. Ptosis
_____	2. Fluid accumulation, swelling	b. Alopecia
_____	3. Loss of hair	c. Edema
_____	4. Drooping of eyelid over the pupil	d. Jaundice
_____	5. Tiny, pinpoint red spots on the skin	e. Bruit
_____	6. Curvature of the thoracic spine	f. Cyanosis
_____	7. Yellow-orange discoloration	g. Kyphosis
_____	8. A hardened area	h. Petechiae
_____	9. Blowing, swishing sound in blood vessel	i. Erythema
_____	10. A red discoloration	j. Induration

Complete the following:

11. Identify the five skills used in physical assessment and briefly describe each.

12. Identify the following positions for physical examination.
    a.

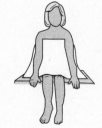

Copyright © 2019, Elsevier Inc. All Rights Reserved.

b.
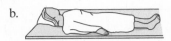

c.
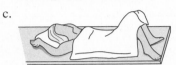

d.
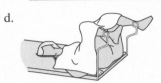

e.
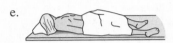

f.
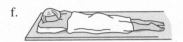

g.
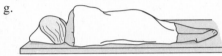

h.
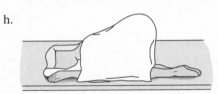

13. Identify which of the pulses is being palpated in each illustration.

a.
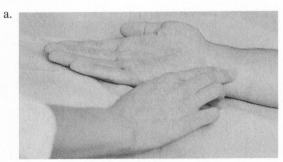

b.
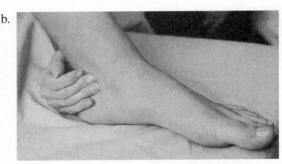

c.
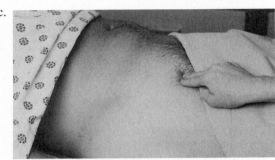

d.
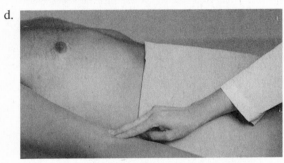

e.
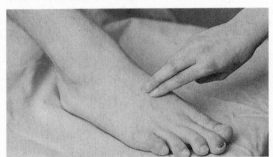

Chapter **16** **Health Assessment and Physical Examination**

Copyright © 2019, Elsevier Inc. All Rights Reserved.

14. Correctly identify the primary skin lesion in each illustration.

a.

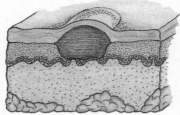

b.

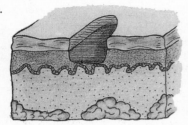

c.

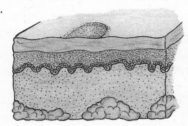

d.

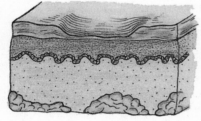

e.

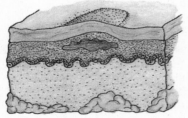

15. Identify on the illustration where the PMI (point of maximal impulse) is located.

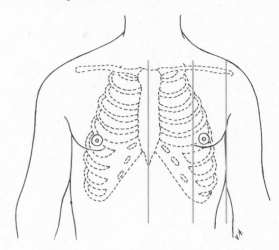

16. Identify both a physical and a behavioral finding that may indicate abuse for each of the following:

	Physical	*Behavioral*
a. Child sexual abuse	_____	_____
b. Intimate partner violence	_____	_____
c. Older adult abuse	_____	_____

17. Identify the abdominal structures that are assessed.
a.

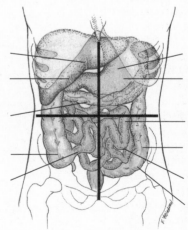

Copyright © 2019, Elsevier Inc. All Rights Reserved.

b.

18. Mark each of the following physical assessment findings as either expected or unexpected. For unexpected findings, investigate what may be the possible etiology.

	Expected	Unexpected
a. Skin lifts easily and snaps back	_____	_____
b. Erythema noted over bony prominences	_____	_____
c. Hair evenly distributed over scalp and pubic area	_____	_____
d. Brown pigmentation of nails in longitudinal streaks (dark-skinned patient)	_____	_____
e. Pallor in face and nail beds	_____	_____
f. Clubbing of nails	_____	_____
g. PEERLA	_____	_____
h. Pupils cloudy	_____	_____
i. Yellow discoloration of sclera	_____	_____
j. Eardrum translucent, shiny, and pearly gray	_____	_____
k. Light brown or gray cerumen	_____	_____
l. Nasal septum midline	_____	_____
m. Nasal mucosa pale with clear, watery discharge	_____	_____
n. Sinuses tender to touch	_____	_____
o. Teeth chalky white, with black discoloration	_____	_____
p. Tongue medium red, moist, and slightly rough on top	_____	_____
q. Soft palate rises when patient says "ah"	_____	_____
r. Uvula reddened and edematous, tonsils with yellow exudate	_____	_____
s. Thyroid gland small, smooth, and free of nodules	_____	_____
t. Lungs resonant to percussion	_____	_____
u. Costal angle greater than 90 degrees between costal margins	_____	_____
v. Bulging of intercostal spaces	_____	_____
w. No carotid bruit present	_____	_____
x. Extra heart sound noted	_____	_____
y. Jugular vein distention at 45-degree angle	_____	_____
z. Dependent edema in ankles	_____	_____
aa. Female breasts smooth, symmetrical, without retraction	_____	_____
bb. Soft, well-differentiated, moveable lumps in the breasts noted	_____	_____
cc. Bowel sounds active and audible in all four quadrants	_____	_____
dd. Bulging flanks	_____	_____
ee. Flat or concave umbilicus	_____	_____
ff. Rebound tenderness found	_____	_____
gg. Perineal skin smooth and slightly darker than surrounding skin	_____	_____
hh. Inguinal bulging	_____	_____
ii. Glans penis smooth and pink on all surfaces	_____	_____
jj. Testes smooth and ovoid	_____	_____
kk. Symmetrical muscle strength	_____	_____
ll. Hips and shoulders aligned parallel	_____	_____
mm. Lordosis of spine noted	_____	_____
nn. Reflexes symmetrical	_____	_____
oo. Unable to repeat series of five numbers	_____	_____

Copyright © 2019, Elsevier Inc. All Rights Reserved.

pp. Able to perform _____ _____
rapidly alternating
movements

qq. Horizontal jerking or _____ _____
bobbing of the head

rr. Positive Romberg test _____ _____

19. A patient has an area of discomfort. The nurse will examine this area:

a. First

b. Last

20. When using the stethoscope, high-pitched sounds are heard best with a:

a. Diaphragm

b. Bell

21. To inspect an adult patient's ear canal, the nurse pulls the auricle:

a. Up and back

b. Down and back

22. The preferred position to place the patient in for a genital examination is:

23. The position to place the patient in for an abdominal examination is:

24. Identify what a nurse is able to assess in a general survey of a patient:

25. What are the general principles for inspection of body areas?

26. What techniques are appropriate when assessing patients of different ages? Select all that apply.
a. Speaking privately with adolescents about their

concerns _____

b. Using closed-end questions to increase the speed

of the examination _____

c. Calling children and their parents by their first

names _____

d. Providing time for children to play _____

e. Performing the examination for an older adult

near bathroom facilities _____

f. Proceeding rapidly through the examination of an older adult to finish it as quickly as possible

_____

27. Patients older than 65 years should be instructed to have yearly eye examinations.

True _____ False _____

28. A nurse is preparing to perform a skin assessment for an average adult patient. Select all of the following techniques that are correct:

a. Using fluorescent lighting _____

b. Keeping the room extremely warm _____

c. Using disposable gloves to inspect lesions _____

d. Looking for coloration changes by checking the

tongue and nail beds _____

29. During a physical examination, a nurse notes that the patient appears to be very anxious. The nurse should:

30. One example of a test for colorectal cancer is:

31. Select the three best positions that a patient may be placed in for a cardiac assessment:

a. Prone _____

b. Supine _____

c. Lithotomy _____

d. Sitting _____

e. Left lateral recumbent _____

f. Dorsal recumbent _____

g. Sims _____

32. Identify signs and symptoms that a patient may have if he or she has cardiopulmonary disease.

33. What are the risk factors associated with osteoporosis? Select all that apply.

a. An active lifestyle _____

b. Smoking _____

c. African American background _____

d. A history of falls _____

e. A history of Cushing disease _____

f. Exposure to sunlight _____

g. A thin, light body frame _____

34. Identify a technique that is used in assessment of the lymph nodes in the head and neck:

Copyright © 2019, Elsevier Inc. All Rights Reserved.

35. Continuous dilation of the pupils is found with the patient experiencing:

36. An expected response when testing the pupils for accommodation is:

37. What is used to weigh the following patients?
    a. Newborn infant
    b. Mobile adult

38. The primary nurse tells the student that the patient is experiencing tinnitus. The student expects that the patient will describe:

39. Three possible causes of hearing loss are:

40. To assess for a pulse deficit, the nurse should:

41. An irregular pulse is counted for _____ seconds.

42. Identify all of the risk factors for breast cancer in a female. Select all that apply.

    a. Under 40 years old _____

    b. Recent use of oral contraceptives _____

    c. Late onset menarche _____

    d. Family history _____

    e. Childless _____

43. The nurse is preparing to do an assessment of the abdomen.
    a. The correct sequence for the abdominal exam is:

    b. Bowel sounds usually occur _____/minute.

    c. What finding is expected for the patient with ascites?

    d. Absent bowel sounds can result from:

44. When teaching the patient about the signs and symptoms of prostate cancer, the nurse should include what information?

45. a. How can the nurse test recent and past memory?

    b. How can abstract thinking be tested?

46. A patient is suspected of substance abuse. What physical findings would be found on the skin? Select all that apply.

    a. Loss of pigment _____

    b. Spider angiomas _____

    c. Hematomas _____

    d. Red, dry areas _____

    e. Burns on the fingers _____

    f. Irregularly shaped moles _____

47. Full range of motion against gravity but not against resistance is noted as grade _____ and _____% normal.

48. Since stethoscopes are used on multiple patients, identify the care that should be provided to promote infection control.

49. If there is a risk or there is evidence of vascular insufficiency, what instruction should be provided to the patient?

50. Which of the following are signs or symptoms of colon cancer? Select all that apply.

    a. Rectal bleeding _____

    b. Tarry stools _____

    c. Nausea _____

    d. Headache _____

    e. Change in bowel pattern _____

    f. Cramping pain in the lower abdomen _____

51. a. How should assessment for skin cancer be done?

    b. Identify at least three instructions to provide patients to help prevent skin cancer.

52. Identify at least three patient behaviors that are "red flags" for suspicion of substance abuse.

53. The nurse is examining the external genitalia of a female patient. When the nurse touches the perineal skin, the patient jumps. What should the nurse have done?

Copyright © 2019, Elsevier Inc. All Rights Reserved.

54. What are the 5 Ps that indicate a vascular occlusion?

55. Provide examples of questions that you should ask during an assessment of the following areas:
    a. Thorax
    b. Abdomen
    c. Musculoskeletal system

56. With _____ a person cannot understand written or verbal speech. With _____ a person understands written and verbal speech but cannot write or speak appropriately when attempting to communicate.

57. You identify that the new intern is palpating both of the carotid arteries at the same time. You point out that this could lead to:

Select the best answer for each of the following questions:

58. A nurse is assessing a patient's nail beds. An expected finding is indicated by:
    1. softening of the nail bed.
    2. a concave curve to the nail.
    3. brown, linear streaks in the nail bed.
    4. a 160-degree angle between the nail plate and nail.

59. A young adult woman arrives at the family planning center for a physical examination. For this patient with mature breasts, the nurse expects to find that the:
    1. breast tissue is softer.
    2. nipples project and areolae have receded.
    3. areolae are dark and have increased diameter.
    4. breasts are elongated and nipples are smaller and flatter.

60. A nurse has checked the medical record and found that a patient has anemia. The presence of anemia is accompanied by the nurse's finding of:
    1. pallor.
    2. erythema.
    3. jaundice.
    4. cyanosis.

61. A patient with asthma has gone to an urgent care center for treatment. On auscultation of the lungs, a nurse hears rhonchi. These sounds are described as:
    1. dry and grating.
    2. loud, low-pitched, and coarse.
    3. high-pitched, fine, and short.
    4. high-pitched and musical.

62. A patient is admitted to a medical center with a peripheral vascular problem. A nurse is performing the initial assessment of the patient. While assessing the lower extremities, the nurse is alert to venous insufficiency as indicated by:
    1. marked edema.
    2. thin, shiny skin.
    3. coolness to touch.
    4. dusky red coloration.

63. A nurse is performing a complete neurological assessment on a patient after a cerebrovascular accident (CVA/stroke). To assess cranial nerve III, the nurse:
    1. uses the Snellen chart.
    2. lightly touches the cornea with a wisp of cotton.
    3. whispers into one ear at a time.
    4. measures pupil reaction to light and accommodation.

64. Student nurses are practicing neurological assessment and determination of cranial nerve functioning. To assess cranial nerve X, the student nurse should ask the patient to:
    1. say "ah."
    2. shrug the shoulders.
    3. smile and frown.
    4. stick out the tongue.

65. While completing a physical examination, a nurse assesses and reports that a patient has petechiae. The nurse has found:
    1. light perspiration on the skin.
    2. moles with regular edges.
    3. thickness on the soles of the feet.
    4. pin-point size, flat, red spots.

66. A nurse reviews a chart and sees that a patient who has been admitted to the unit this morning has a hyperthyroid disorder. The nurse anticipates that an examination of the eyes will reveal:
    1. diplopia.
    2. strabismus.
    3. exophthalmos.
    4. nystagmus.

67. In preparation for an examination of the internal ear, a nurse anticipates that the color of the eardrum should appear:
    1. white.
    2. yellow.
    3. slightly red.
    4. pearly gray.

67

Copyright © 2019, Elsevier Inc. All Rights Reserved.

68. A patient with a history of smoking and alcohol abuse has gone to a clinic for a physical examination. Based on this history, the nurse is particularly alert during an examination of the oral cavity to the presence of:
   1. thick, white patches.
   2. spongy gums.
   3. pink tissue.
   4. loose teeth.

69. A patient in a physician's office has an increased anteroposterior diameter of the chest. The nurse should inquire specifically about the patient's history of:
   1. lung disease.
   2. thoracic trauma.
   3. spinal surgery.
   4. exposure to hepatitis.

70. When auscultating a patient's chest, a nurse hears what appears to be an S₃ sound. This is an expected finding if the patient is:
   1. 10 years old.
   2. 35 years old.
   3. 56 years old.
   4. 82 years old.

71. A patient in a medical center has been prescribed bed rest for a prolonged period of time. There is a possibility that the patient may have developed phlebitis. The nurse assesses for the presence of this condition by:
   1. palpating the ankles for pitting edema.
   2. checking the popliteal pulses bilaterally.
   3. inspecting the thighs for clusters of ecchymosis.
   4. checking the appearance and circumference of the lower legs.

72. A sweet, fruity odor on the breath is associated with:
   1. bronchial infection.
   2. poor oral hygiene.
   3. diabetic ketoacidosis.
   4. malabsorption syndrome.

73. A patient has been experiencing some lightheadedness and loss of balance over the past few weeks. A nurse wants to check the patient's balance while waiting for the patient to have other laboratory tests. The nurse administers the:
   1. Allen test.
   2. Rinne test.
   3. Weber test.
   4. Romberg test.

74. Screenings are being conducted at the junior high school for scoliosis. A nurse is observing the students for the presence of:
   1. an S-shaped curvature of the spine.
   2. an exaggerated curvature of the thoracic spine.
   3. an exaggerated curvature of the lumbar spine.
   4. a bulging of the cervical vertebrae and disks.

75. While reviewing a medical record, a nurse notes that a patient has suspected pancreatitis. The nurse assesses the patient for:
   1. positive rebound tenderness.
   2. midline abdominal pulsations.
   3. hyperactive bowel sounds in all quadrants.
   4. bulging of the flanks with dependent distention.

76. An 80-year-old woman is being assessed by a nurse in an extended care facility. The nurse is assessing the genitalia of this patient and suspects that there may be a malignancy present. The nurse's suspicion is due to the finding of:
   1. scaly, nodular lesions.
   2. yellow exudates and redness.
   3. small ulcers with serous drainage.
   4. extreme pallor and edema.

77. A screening for osteoporosis is being conducted at an annual health fair. To determine the risk factors for osteoporosis, a nurse is assessing individuals for:
   1. multiparity.
   2. a heavier than recommended body frame.
   3. an African American background.
   4. a history of dieting and/or alcohol abuse.

78. A patient in a rehabilitation facility has experienced a cerebrovascular accident (CVA/stroke) that has left the patient with an expressive aphasia. The nurse anticipates that this patient will:
   1. be unable to speak or write.
   2. be unable to follow directions.
   3. respond appropriately to questions.
   4. have difficulty interpreting words and phrases.

79. To assess a patient's visual fields, a nurse should:
   1. ask the patient to read text.
   2. turn the room light on and off.
   3. move a finger at arm's length toward the patient from an angle.
   4. shine a penlight into the patient's eye at an oblique angle.

80. A nurse exerts downward pressure on the thigh and asks the patient to raise the leg up. This assessment is determining the muscle strength of the:
   1. triceps.
   2. trapezius.
   3. quadriceps.
   4. gastrocnemius.

81. Light palpation involves depressing the part being examined:
   1. ½ inch.
   2. 1 inch.
   3. 1½ inches.
   4. 2 inches.

Copyright © 2019, Elsevier Inc. All Rights Reserved.

82. A nurse teaches the male patient that he should notify a health care provider if he finds the following during a testicular self-examination:
    1. loose, deeper color scrotal skin with a coarse surface.
    2. cordlike structures on the top of the testicles.
    3. small, pea-sized lumps on the front of the testicle.
    4. smegma under the foreskin.

83. A nurse manager observes a new nurse on the unit performing a patient assessment. The new nurse's assessment should be interrupted if the manager observes the nurse:
    1. using the pads of the first three fingers to palpate the breast tissue.
    2. auscultating the abdomen continuously for 5 minutes.
    3. palpating both carotid arteries simultaneously.
    4. testing sensory function on random locations with the patient's eyes closed.

84. A nurse assesses a patient's skin and documents that vesicles are present. This observation is based on the nurse finding:
    1. flat, nonpalpable changes in skin color.
    2. palpable, solid elevations smaller than 1 cm.
    3. irregularly shaped, elevated areas that vary in size.
    4. circumscribed elevations of skin filled with serous fluid.

85. A nurse is assessing a patient's level of consciousness using the Glasgow Coma Scale. The following findings are documented: Eyes open to speech, responses are oriented, localized pain is noted. The score for this patient is:
    1. 15.
    2. 13.
    3. 11.
    4. 9.

86. To assess the temperature of the patient's skin, the nurse should use the:
    1. thumbs.
    2. fingertips
    3. palm of the hand.
    4. dorsal surface of the hand.

87. The patient needs to sit upright in order to breathe easier. This is recorded by the nurse as:
    1. apnea.
    2. dyspnea.
    3. orthopnea.
    4. tachypnea.

STUDY GROUP QUESTIONS

- What are the purposes of the physical examination?
- How is physical assessment integrated into patient care?
- How does a nurse incorporate cultural sensitivity and awareness of ethnic physiological differences into the physical examination?
- What are the physical assessment skills, and what information is obtained through their use?
- How does a nurse prepare a patient and environment for a physical examination?
- What similarities and differences exist in the preparation and procedure for a physical examination of a child, adult, and older adult?
- What information is obtained through a general survey?
- What positions and equipment are used for completion of the physical examination?
- What is the usual sequence for performing the physical examination?
- Which nursing history information should be obtained while proceeding through the physical examination?
- What are the expected and unexpected findings of a complete physical examination?
- What self-screening procedures may be taught to patients?
- How does a nurse report and record the findings of a physical examination?

STUDY CHART

Create a study chart to identify specific abnormalities to be alert for in each body system, working in sequential order of the exam from the integumentary system through the neurological system.

Copyright © 2019, Elsevier Inc. All Rights Reserved.

Medication Administration

PRELIMINARY READING

Chapter 17, pp. 379–478

CASE STUDIES

1. You are visiting a patient at home who has poor eyesight and occasional forgetfulness. The patient has four oral medications to take at different times of the day. He tells you that he doesn't think that he can remember to take them all and that he can't remember what information he was given by the prescriber.
   a. What strategies may be implemented to assist this patient in maintaining the medication regimen?

2. You are preparing to give medications to a patient in a long-term care facility, but the prescriber's handwriting is difficult to read.
   a. What should you do to prevent medication errors?

3. A patient in a long-term care facility is about to receive her medications, but you notice that she does not have an identification band.
   a. What is the appropriate next action?

4. You are going to administer an injection to a 6-year-old child on a pediatric acute care unit.
   a. What safety measures should you implement?

5. The patient has just received an immunization and appears to be having an anaphylactic reaction.
   a. What treatments are anticipated?

6. You are about to prepare a narcotic medication for administration to a patient. The record shows that 24 tablets should remain in the box but there are only 23 tablets left.
   a. What should you do?

7. You are caring for a patient who requires an antipyretic medication that is ordered for oral administration, but the patient has been experiencing severe nausea.
   a. What are your actions?

Copyright © 2019, Elsevier Inc. All Rights Reserved.

CHAPTER REVIEW

Match the description/definition in Column A with the correct term in Column B.

Column A

_____ 1. Placing medication under the tongue

_____ 2. The effect of two medications combined is greater than each given separately

_____ 3. Secondary effects of medication, such as nausea

_____ 4. Unpredictable effect of medications

_____ 5. Fluid administered and retained in a body cavity

_____ 6. Injection into tissues below the dermis of the skin

_____ 7. Severe allergic response characterized by bronchospasm and laryngeal edema

_____ 8. Inserting medication into the eye

_____ 9. Administering medications through the oral, nasal, or pulmonary passages

_____ 10. Patient taking many medications

_____ 11. Placing solid medication against the mucous membranes of the cheek

_____ 12. Injecting medication into body tissues

Column B

a. Parenteral administration

b. Inhalation

c. Instillation

d. Buccal

e. Subcutaneous

f. Intraocular

g. Idiosyncratic reaction

h. Polypharmacy

i. Sublingual

j. Synergistic effect

k. Side effects

l. Anaphylactic reaction

Complete the following:

13. Provide an example of how a nurse's professional responsibility in administering medications is controlled or regulated.

14. a. Identify a strategy for a nurse to implement to avoid errors with medications that appear the same.

    b. Specify two acceptable patient identifiers.

15. Provide an example of how each of the following factors can influence the actions of medications.
    a. Dietary factors
    b. Physiological variables
    c. Environmental conditions

16. Identify the four routes for parenteral administration of medications.

17. For the following medication orders, identify the essential component that is missing. (NOTE: All are for the correct patient and have been signed by the prescriber.)
    a. Apresoline IM stat
    b. Morphine sulfate 10 mg q3-4h
    c. Vancomycin 1 g IV
    d. Lasix 40 mg bid

18. Identify the six guidelines or "rights" that a nurse uses for administering medications.

    1. _____
    2. _____
    3. _____
    4. _____
    5. _____
    6. _____

19. Place the following steps for removing medication from a vial for an IM injection in the correct sequence:

    a. Select the correct needle and syringe _____

    b. Dislodge air bubbles _____

    c. Insert the needle through the rubber seal of the vial _____

    d. Remove the syringe from the vial _____

    e. Perform hand hygiene _____

    f. Inject the air in the syringe into the air space in the vial. _____

    g. Remove the needle cap _____

    h. Pull back on the plunger of the syringe and withdraw air equal to the volume of medication to be administered _____

Copyright © 2019, Elsevier Inc. All Rights Reserved.

i. Invert the vial and fill the syringe to the correct volume of medication _____

j. Remove the cap from the vial _____

20. Identify the form of medication for the following.
    a. Solid dose form for oral use; medication in a powder, liquid, or oil form and encased by a gelatin shell:
    b. Solid dose form mixed with gelatin and shaped in form of pellet for insertion into body cavity:
    c. Clear liquid containing water and/or alcohol; designed for oral use; usually has a sweetener added:
    d. Finely divided drug particles dispersed in a liquid medium; when left standing, particles settle to the bottom of the container:
    e. Semiliquid suspension used to cool, protect, or clean the skin:

21. a. An example of a commonly abused prescription medication is:

    b. An example of a commonly abused over-the-counter medication is:

22. Adherence to medication therapy:
    a. Noncompliance with or nonadherence to medication therapy may be related to:

    b. Identify at least one strategy to promote medication adherence.

23. MedWatch is a _____
    _____.

24. For each of the following pairs, identify which of the two has the faster absorption or action in the body:
    a. IV _____   or   Oral _____
    b. IM _____   or   Subcutaneous _____
    c. Acidic oral   or   Alkaline oral
       medication _____   medication _____
    d. Tablets _____   or   Solutions _____
    e. Larger surface   or   Smaller surface area
       area _____   _____
    f. Less lipid   or   Highly lipid soluble
       soluble _____   _____
    g. Albumin binding   or   Nonalbumin binding
       z   _____

25. The time that it takes for a medication to reach its highest effective concentration is its:

26. Oral medication is contraindicated for a patient with:

27. What is a potential problem with these medication orders?
    a. Lasix 40.0 mg

    b. Digoxin .25 mg

28. Identify the appropriate equivalents for the following:
    a. 1 ounce = _____ mL
    b. 60 mL = _____ ounces
    c. _____ L = 1 quart
    d. 3 g = _____ mg
    e. 0.25 L = _____ mL
    f. _____ mL = 1 teaspoon

29. For medication orders:
    a. Identify the five different types of medication orders and provide an example of each:
       1.
       2.
       3.
       4.
       5.

30. Verbal orders are usually required to be signed by the prescriber within what time frame?

31. A nurse calculates the medication order and determines that 6 tablets should be given to the patient for each dose. What should the nurse do first?

32. Describe the difference between an adverse and a side effect.

33. a. The nurse is preparing to give medications and the patient says that the medicine looks different from the previous administrations of the medication. The nurse should:

    b. The patient refuses a medication that the nurse is preparing to administer. The nurse should:

Copyright © 2019, Elsevier Inc. All Rights Reserved.

34. Identify the correct techniques for medication administration. Select all that apply.
    a. Discarding the patient's unopened unit-dose medication that was refused. _____
    b. Crushing medication and mixing it in a large amount of food to mask the taste. _____
    c. Noting in the record if a patient refuses a medication. _____
    d. Recording medications before administration. _____
    e. Giving another nurse's medications to the patient. _____
    f. Administering non-time-critical medications within 1-2 hours of the scheduled time. _____
    g. Aspirating when giving immunizations. _____
    h. Documenting the patient's response in the record. _____

35. Identify the generic names for the following drugs:
    a. Levaquin
    b. Lasix
    c. Advil
    d. Haldol

36. A triple check to compare the medication label to the order should be done:
    1.
    2.
    3.

37. Identify a technique that may be used to facilitate administration of medications to children.
    a. Oral medications:
    b. Injections:

38. Identify a way that a nurse may minimize the discomfort of an injection.

39. How should a medication that is irritating to the tissues be injected?

40. Identify the correct angle for each of the following illustrations, and the type of injection that is being administered.

    a. _____   b. _____   c. _____

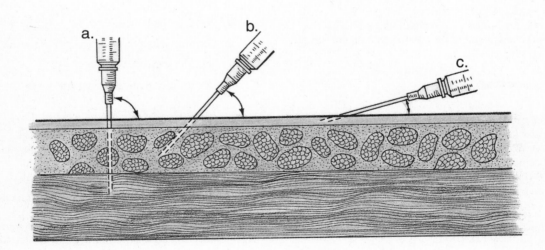

41. Identify three ways in which medication may be administered intravenously.
    a.
    b.
    c.

42. A wireless barcode scanner is usually used to identify:
    a.
    b.
    c.

Copyright © 2019, Elsevier Inc. All Rights Reserved.

43. Identify the meaning of the following abbreviations.

a. ac: _____

b. bid: _____

c. prn: _____

d. q4h: _____

e. stat: _____

44. Check the orders and calculate the correct dosages for the following medication orders.

a. Prescriber's order: Synthroid 0.150 mg PO daily
   In stock: Split tablets in a container labeled 75 mcg
   How many tablets should be given?

b. Prescriber's order: Prilosec 40 mg PO bid
   In stock: Prilosec 20 mg tablets
   How much of the medication should be given?

c. Prescriber's order: Lasix 20 mg IM stat
   In stock: Lasix 10 mg/mL
   How much medication should be given?

d. Prescriber's order: hydrocortisone succinate 200 mg/day in two equal doses
   In stock: hydrocortisone succinate 50 mg/mL
   How much medication should be given for each dose?
   Mark the amount to be administered on the syringe.

e. Prescriber's order: Regular insulin 24 units
   In stock: Regular insulin U-100
   How much medication should be administered?
   Mark the amount to be administered on the syringe.

f. Prescriber's order: Cefazolin 500 mg q8h
   In stock: Keflex 250 mg tablets
   How many tablets should be given?

g. The medication is mixed in 50 mL of fluid in a volume-controlled set and will be infused with a minidrip (60 gtt/mL) over 1 hour.

   The nurse sets the rate to infuse at: _____ drops/minute

h. Prescriber's order: Xanax 0.5 mg tid.
   In stock: Xanax 1 mg scored tablets
   How much should be given for each administration?

45. Identify an area of patient assessment before administration of a parenteral injection.

46. Identify on the figure the sites recommended for subcutaneous injections.

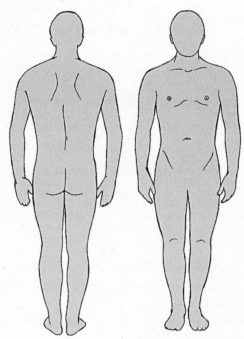

47. Select all of the following actions that are correct to prevent aspiration when administering medications to a patient with dysphagia.

a. Do not allow the patient to self-administer, even if able. _____

b. Position the patient upright. _____

c. Turn the patient's head toward the weaker side to help the patient swallow. _____

d. Use thinner liquids for the patient to take with the medications. _____

e. Use a straw for liquids. _____

f. Crush medication and mix with pureed food, if indicated. _____

48. For medication administration through a nasogastric tube:

a. A priority assessment specifically for the patient receiving medication through a nasogastric tube is for the nurse to:

b. How should the patient be positioned, if possible?

c. The tube should be flushed with _____ mL of _____ in between each medication, and flushed after all medications are given with _____ mL.

d. How should tablets be administered?

Copyright © 2019, Elsevier Inc. All Rights Reserved.

49. Before administration of a topical medication, the nurse needs to:

50. Identify the following for the administration of ear medication:
    a. Position the patient:

    b. Pull ear pinna _____ for an adult patient.

    c. Irrigate with _____ mL of _____ temperature fluid.

51. For the use of a pressured metered-dose inhaler (pMDI):
    a. When the patient has difficulty coordinating the inhaler, a(n) _____ should be used.

    b. The patient should inhale for _____ seconds while pressing down on the canister and hold the breath for _____ seconds.

    c. How much time should be given in between administration of the same medication?

    d. The medication order is 2 puffs of the inhaler qid. The canister contains 160 puffs total.
       How many days will the canister last?

       _____

    e. Following the administration of a steroid inhalation, the patient should:

52. a. The patient should be placed in _____ position for the administration of a rectal suppository.

    b. How do you prepare the suppository?

    c. How far is the suppository inserted for an adult _____ or child _____.

53. The correct way to expel air from the syringe is to:

54. a. Eye drops should be administered directly onto the cornea.

       True _____ False _____

    b. A nurse is responsible for administering an incorrect medication or dosage.

       True _____ False _____

    c. You do not need to aspirate when giving intradermal or subcutaneous injections.

       True _____ False _____

    d. Misuse and abuse of prescription drugs occur more often than other drugs, except marijuana and alcohol.

       True _____ False _____

55. From the following, identify the guidelines that are appropriate for pediatric medication administration. Select all that apply.
    a. Identify the dosage based on the child's weight in pounds. _____

    b. Pediatric doses are usually given in micrograms and small syringes. _____

    c. IM doses are very small and usually do not exceed 1 mL in small children. _____

    d. Most medications are rounded to the nearest tenth. _____

    e. Mentally estimate a patient's dose before beginning the calculation, comparing the answer with the estimate before preparing the medication. _____

    f. Dosage ranges for 24-hour periods are similar to adult dosages. _____

56. Identify the correct sequence of actions for a saline flush.
    a. Pulling back gently on syringe plunger and checking for blood return _____

    b. Cleaning lock's injection port with antiseptic swab _____

    c. Flushing IV site with normal saline by pushing slowly on plunger _____

    d. Removing saline-filled syringe _____

    e. Preparing two syringes filled with 2–3 mL of normal saline (0.9%) _____

    f. Inserting syringe with normal saline 0.9% through injection port of IV lock _____

57. During an IM injection, blood is aspirated. The nurse should:

58. For IV push or bolus medication administration:
    a. The medication should be infused at a rate of 2 mL over 2 minutes: this is how many mL every 30 seconds? _____.

    b. If the medication is incompatible with the IV fluid that is infusing, the nurse should:

59. Identify the sites that may be used for an intradermal injection.

Copyright © 2019, Elsevier Inc. All Rights Reserved.

60. A tuberculin test has been administered.

    a. Results should be read in _____ hours.

    b. A positive test for an individual with no known risk factors is: _____.

61. The patient is to receive a vaginal cream medication.

    a. The preferred position is: _____.

    b. The applicator is inserted: _____ cm or _____ inches.

    c. After administration, have the patient:

62. Provide examples of beneficial and negative synergistic effects.

63. An advantage of computerized physician order entry to medications is:

64. When do medication orders need to be rewritten by the prescriber?

65. What safety measures are used when withdrawing medication from an ampule?

66. The patient needs to have multiple subcutaneous injections. The basic rule for site rotation is to:

67. Place the steps for administration of an oral medication in the correct order.

    a. Label the medication cups. _____

    b. Compare the medication with the MAR (Medication Administration Record). _____

    c. Identify the patient. _____

    d. Place the unit doses into the cups. _____

    e. Perform hand hygiene. _____

    f. Compare the prepared medication with the MAR. _____

    g. Obtain the medications from the patient's drawer. _____

68. Identify how each of the following may be influenced.
    a. Absorption:
    b. Membrane permeability:
    c. Excretion:

69. The patient tells you that he has an allergy to a particular drug. What are your next actions?

70. The medication order is for 50 mg. The medication comes as 100 mg/mL. Based upon this information, you can estimate that you will give more or less than a mL?

71. How do automated medication dispensing systems generally function?

72. a. You have given the wrong medication to a patient. What are your next actions?

    b. The health care provider orders "Lasix 400 mg po daily."
       • Should you administer this medication?
       • If not, what should you do?

73. What are the benefits and disadvantages/contraindications of the following route?

Route	Benefits	Disadvantages/ Contraindications
Inhalation		

74. Which of the following interventions will assist in preventing medication errors? Select all that apply.

    a. Prepare medications for all of your patients at once to save time. _____

    b. Check labels two times before administering medications. _____

    c. Use at least two patient identifiers. _____

    d. Document all medications as soon as they are given. _____

    e. Follow institution policies and procedures when using technology. _____

    f. Interpret illegible handwriting to the best of your ability. _____

75. Identify at least five of the best practices for administration of IV solutions and medications.

76. How is ophthalmic ointment administered?

77. A nurse *never* prepares which high-alert medications on a patient care unit?

Copyright © 2019, Elsevier Inc. All Rights Reserved.

78. Identify the landmarks for a deltoid IM injection.

Select the best answer for each of the following questions:

79. A nurse determines the location for an injection by identifying the greater trochanter of the femur, anterior superior iliac spine, and iliac crest. The injection site being used by the nurse is the:
    1. rectus femoris muscle.
    2. ventrogluteal area.
    3. dorsogluteal area.
    4. vastus lateralis muscle.

80. Upon receiving the assignment for the evening, a nurse notices that two of the patients have the same name. The best way to identify two patients on a medical unit who have the same name is to:
    1. ask the patients their names.
    2. verify their names with the family members.
    3. check the patients' ID bands and patient information.
    4. ask another nurse about their identities.

81. A nurse is to administer a subcutaneous injection to an average-size adult. The nurse selects a:
    1. 27-gauge, ½-inch needle and 0.5-mL syringe.
    2. 25-gauge, ⅝-inch needle and 1-mL syringe.
    3. 22-gauge, 1-inch needle and 3-mL syringe.
    4. 20-gauge, 1-inch needle and 3-mL syringe.

82. A nurse has administered medications to all assigned patients on the medical unit. Upon assessing the response of the medications given, the nurse is alert to the possibility of a toxic reaction. This is indicated by the patient experiencing:
    1. itching.
    2. nausea.
    3. dizziness.
    4. respiratory depression.

83. The nursing staff is completing a review of the procedures used for the storage and administration of narcotics. A nurse implements the required procedure when:
    1. narcotics are kept together with the patient's other medications.
    2. small amounts of medication may be discarded without notation.
    3. the narcotic count is checked daily by the medication nurse.
    4. a separate inventory record is used to keep an ongoing count.

84. The patient has nose drops ordered that need to reach the posterior pharynx. The patient should be positioned supine with the head:
    1. straight.
    2. tilted backwards.
    3. tilted over the edge of the bed.
    4. bent back over a pillow with the head turned to the side.

85. Which of the following abbreviations is appropriate to use?
    1. hs
    2. SC
    3. qh
    4. TIW

86. A patient in a nurse practitioner's office is receiving penicillin for the first time. The nurse asks the patient to wait in the office following the administration of the medication. The nurse is observing for a possible anaphylactic response that would be demonstrated by:
    1. drowsiness.
    2. dyspnea.
    3. an increased blood pressure reading.
    4. a decreased temperature.

87. A drug that is to be given on a q4h schedule may be administered at:
    1. 10 a.m. and 10 p.m.
    2. 10 a.m., 2 p.m., and 10 p.m.
    3. 10 a.m., 2 p.m., 6 p.m., and 10 p.m.
    4. 10 a.m., 2 p.m., 6 p.m., 10 p.m., and 2 a.m.

88. A specific assessment that a nurse should make before the administration of an anticoagulant is to check for:
    1. an allergy history.
    2. evidence of bruising or bleeding.
    3. the patient's level of discomfort.
    4. increased blood pressure.

89. In the event of a mistake in the administration of medications, the first action that a nurse should take is to:
    1. complete an occurrence report.
    2. inform the patient of the problem.
    3. report the error to the nurse in charge or the physician.
    4. provide an appropriate antidote for the medication given.

90. The subcutaneous site that is most commonly used for low molecular weight heparin injections is the:
    1. abdomen.
    2. anterior thigh.
    3. scapular region.
    4. outer aspect of the upper arm.

91. A prescriber indicates to a nurse that a patient will be receiving an intermediate-acting insulin. The nurse anticipates that the patient will receive:
    1. insulin glargine (Lantus).
    2. insulin lispro (Humalog).
    3. isophane insulin suspension (NPH).
    4. protamine zinc insulin suspension (PZI).

Copyright © 2019, Elsevier Inc. All Rights Reserved.

92. A charge nurse is evaluating the injection technique of a new staff member. The correct technique for a Z-track injection is noted when the new staff member:
    1. uses the deltoid site.
    2. pulls the skin 1 to 1½ inches laterally.
    3. removes the needle immediately after the injection.
    4. releases the skin before the needle is removed.

93. For a subcutaneous injection to an average size adult, which of the following techniques requires correction? The student nurse:
    1. selects a 25-gauge, ⅝-inch needle.
    2. injects the needle at a 45-degree angle.
    3. recaps the needle after injecting the medication.
    4. does not massage the injection site after administration.

94. A nurse is aware that a parenteral administration of medication in a small bag of fluid (25–250 mL) is a:
    1. bolus injection.
    2. piggyback infusion.
    3. primary infusion.
    4. volume-control administration.

95. The patient who will most likely have difficulty with the excretion of medication from the body is the individual who has:
    1. diabetes mellitus.
    2. renal failure.
    3. circulatory insufficiency.
    4. Parkinson's disease.

96. Which prescriber's order takes priority when preparing medications?
    1. PRN
    2. Now
    3. Stat
    4. Standing

97. The patient appears to be having a mild allergic reaction to a medication and is experiencing itching of the skin. This is documented by the nurse as:
    1. urticaria.
    2. rash.
    3. pruritus.
    4. rhinitis.

98. The medication that the patient is taking is ototoxic. Based on this information, the nurse knows to specifically assess the patient's:
    1. respiratory rate.
    2. urinary output.
    3. blood pressure.
    4. hearing.

99. The recommended amount of IM medication that can be given safely at one time to an average-sized older adult is:
    1. 0.5 mL.
    2. 1 mL.
    3. 2 mL.
    4. 3 mL.

100. If the medication has been administered after meals, the nurse will document that it has been given:
    1. PC.
    2. prn.
    3. q a.m.
    4. daily.

STUDY GROUP QUESTIONS

- How are medications named and classified, and what forms of medications are available?
- What legislation and standards guide medication administration?
- How are medications absorbed, distributed, metabolized, and excreted from the body?
- What are the different types of medication actions?
- What are the different routes for medication administration, and what are the advantages, disadvantages, and contraindications for each route?
- What are the systems used for drug measurement, and how are amounts converted within and between the systems?
- How are dosages calculated for oral, parenteral, and pediatric medications?
- What are the roles of the health team members in the administration of medications?
- What are the six "rights" of medication administration?
- What patient assessment data are critical to obtain before administering medications?
- What equipment is used for the administration of medications via different routes?
- What are the sites or body landmarks for parenteral administration?
- What are the procedures for administration of medications?
- How can IV medication be administered?
- How is administration of medications adapted to patients of different ages and levels of health?
- What information is included in patient/family teaching for medication administration?
- How has technology influenced the administration of medications?

STUDY CHART

Create a study chart to compare *Parenteral Medication and Preparation* that identifies the equipment, needle gauge, amount of medication, site to be used, and angle of injection for subcutaneous, intramuscular, and intradermal injections.

Copyright © 2019, Elsevier Inc. All Rights Reserved.

18 Fluid, Electrolyte, and Acid-Base Balances

PRELIMINARY READING

Chapter 18, pp. 479–535

CASE STUDIES

1. The patient is diagnosed with heart failure and will be taking digoxin and Lasix on a daily basis.
   a. What patient teaching is indicated in relation to possible fluid and electrolyte imbalances?

2. You are working with two patients today. One of the patients is unconscious and is experiencing a period of prolonged immobility. The other patient has a long history of alcoholism. You are alert to possible alterations in fluid and electrolyte imbalance.
   a. What specific signs and symptoms may these patients exhibit as a result of their present conditions?

3. An adult male patient has come to the outpatient clinic for an examination. During the initial interview, the patient tells you that he has smoked 2½ packs of cigarettes each day for the last 25 years.
   a. What physical signs do you anticipate finding because of the patient's history?
   b. What acid-base imbalance is this patient most likely to experience?

4. Following a motor vehicle accident, the patient had traumatic injuries and a significant hemorrhage. He will be receiving blood transfusions.
   a. What are the priority assessments that should be completed prior to administration of the blood?
   b. What safety measures should be implemented to reduce the possibility of complications?

CHAPTER REVIEW

Match the description/definition in Column A with the correct term in Column B.

Column A	Column B
_____ 1. Positively charged electrolytes	a. Anions
_____ 2. Having the same osmotic pressure	b. Diffusion
_____ 3. Movement of water across a semipermeable membrane	c. Filtration
_____ 4. Movement of molecules from an area of higher concentration to an area of lower concentration	d. Active transport
_____ 5. Negatively charged electrolytes	e. Cations
_____ 6. Movement of solutes out of a solution with greater hydrostatic pressure	f. Isotonic
_____ 7. A compound that separates into ions when dissolved in water	g. Hypotonic
_____ 8. Overall particle concentration	h. Osmosis
_____ 9. Having a lower osmotic pressure	i. Osmolality
_____ 10. Movement of molecules to an area of higher concentration	j. Electrolyte

Copyright © 2019, Elsevier Inc. All Rights Reserved.

Complete the following:

11. Identify the following terms:
    a. All fluids outside of the cell:
    b. Fluid between the cells and outside the blood vessels (within tissues):
    c. All fluids within the cell:

12. Identify if the following electrolytes are cations or anions, whether they are primarily extracellular or intracellular, and their primary role in the body:
    a. Sodium:
    b. Potassium:
    c. Calcium:
    d. Magnesium:
    e. Chloride:
    f. Bicarbonate:
    g. Phosphate:

13. Acid-base balance in the body is regulated by:

14. What age groups are most susceptible to fluid and acid-base imbalances?

15. Identify whether the following solutions are isotonic, hypertonic, or hypotonic:
    a. Dextrose 5% in water (D5W):
    b. 0.45% sodium chloride (0.45% NS):
    c. 0.9% sodium chloride (0.9% NS):
    d. Lactated Ringer's (LR):
    e. Dextrose 5% in 0.45% sodium chloride:

16. Identify three types of medications that may cause fluid, electrolyte, or acid-base imbalances.

17. Specify two possible nursing diagnoses for patients experiencing fluid, electrolyte, or acid-base imbalances.

18. Identify the sites for an IV infusion.

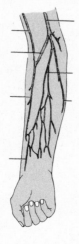

19. A patient who is NPO, with normal renal function, needs to have _____ added to the solution.

20. Identify the signs and symptoms that are associated with phlebitis at an IV site.

21. A patient with a peripherally inserted central catheter (PICC) line develops a fever and increased white blood cell (WBC) count. The nurse anticipates that the health care provider will order:

22. The patient had a rapid infusion of IV fluids and has developed crackles in the lungs, shortness of breath, and tachycardia. The nurse should:

23. Transfusion of a patient's own blood is termed:

24. Identify the electrolyte imbalance that is associated with each of the following test results:
    a. Serum sodium level—125 mEq/L:
    b. Serum potassium level—5.8 mEq/L:
    c. Serum ionized calcium level—3.7 mEq/L:
    d. Serum magnesium level—1.2 mEq/L:

25. Calculate the following IV infusion rates:
    a. IV 500 mL of D_5W to infuse in 5 hours; drop factor = 15 gtt/mL. How many gtt/min should be infused?
    b. IV 1000 mL of NS to infuse in 8 hours; drop factor = 10 gtt/mL. How many gtt/min should be infused?
    c. IV 200 mL of NS to infuse in 4 hours; drop factor = 60 gtt/mL. How many gtt/min should be infused?
    d. IV 2 L of D_5W to infuse in 18 hours. How many ml/hour should be set on the infusion pump?

26. Identify the hormones that control fluid balance:

27. If a hypotonic solution is given intravenously to a patient, the fluid will move into the cells.

    True _____ False _____

28. Arterial pH is an indirect measurement of:

29. What aspect of intake and output is usually able to be delegated to NAP?

30. An average adult's daily total intake of fluid is approximately _____ mL.

Copyright © 2019, Elsevier Inc. All Rights Reserved.

31. The nurse is going to perform a venipuncture in order to initiate IV therapy. Place the following steps in the correct order:

    a. Prepare the IV infusion tubing and solution _____

    b. Reapply the tourniquet _____

    c. Perform hand hygiene _____

    d. Cleanse the site _____

    e. Select a large-enough vein _____

32. The nurse is calculating the patient's intake and output for the last 8 hours. During this time, the patient consumed 1 cup of gelatin, ½ cup of juice, 1 cup of water, and 1 cup of tea. The IV infusion started with 750 mL in the bag, with 125 mL remaining at the end of the shift. The urinary output was 340 mL and there was 30 mL of drainage from the nasogastric tube.
    Cup = 8 oz
    What is the patient's intake and output?

    I = _____   O = _____

33. Which of the following is/are most likely to lead to a fluid volume deficit? Select all that apply.

    a. Vomiting _____

    b. Heart failure _____

    c. Corticosteroid administration _____

    d. Fever _____

    e. Increased sodium intake _____

    f. Diuretic administration _____

34. A patient has a nursing diagnosis of *insufficient fluid volume related to excessive diaphoresis* from fever. Identify a related outcome and two nursing interventions for this patient:

35. When selecting a site to start an IV, the nurse should begin with the site that is: _____

36. The IV site is located in the right antecubital space. The nurse notes that the rate fluctuates when the patient flexes his right arm. The nurse should:

37. Identify the correct order of the following steps for the removal of an IV.

    a. Turn off the roller clamp _____

    b. Remove the IV catheter _____

    c. Remove the dressing _____

    d. Record the fluid infusion _____

    e. Inspect the tip of the IV catheter _____

    f. Perform hand hygiene and apply clean gloves _____

    g. Place gauze over the site and apply light pressure _____

38. The nurse is preparing the IV fluid infusion.
    a. What should be checked when looking at the IV fluid?

    b. When is venipuncture contraindicated for a site?

39. a. In preparing to administer a blood transfusion, what are the critical assessments that need to be made?

    b. What is the usual infusion time for a unit of blood? What is the maximum length of time that blood should be allowed to infuse?

40. It is suspected that the patient is experiencing hypokalemia. Identify all of the signs that support this assessment. Select all that apply.

    a. Bilateral muscle weakness _____

    b. Positive Chvostek's sign _____

    c. Bradycardia _____

    d. Diminished bowel sounds _____

    e. Tetany _____

    f. ECG abnormalities _____

41. Identify which of the following are correct when performing an IV site dressing. Select all that apply.

    a. Apply tape over the IV insertion site _____

    b. Cleanse the site _____

    c. Use skin protectant where the tape will be _____

    d. Anchor the IV tubing _____

    e. Use clean technique for the procedure _____

    f. Use a catheter stabilization device _____

Copyright © 2019, Elsevier Inc. All Rights Reserved.

42. Which of the following are expected when assessing a patient with ECV excess? Select all that apply.

    a. Hypotension _____

    b. Bounding pulse _____

    c. Dependent edema _____

    d. Thirst _____

    e. Slow capillary refill _____

    f. Distended neck veins when upright _____

43. Identify at least three ways to decrease intravascular infection related to intravenous therapy (IV).

44. Unless specified differently in agency policy, IVs should be monitored q _____ h.

45. Indicate precautions for venipuncture in an older adult patient:

Select the best answer for each of the following questions:

46. The IV site is swollen, pale, and cool to the touch. The nurse identifies this as:
    1. phlebitis.
    2. infiltration.
    3. local infection.
    4. allergic response.

47. A hypotonic IV solution is expected to be administered to a patient who is experiencing:
    1. hypernatremia.
    2. hypocalcemia.
    3. hypervolemia.
    4. hypokalemia.

48. The patient has hypernatremia with a fluid deficit. The nurse anticipates finding:
    1. dry mucous membranes.
    2. orthostatic hypotension.
    3. abdominal cramping.
    4. diarrhea.

49. The patient who is experiencing a gastrointestinal problem has had periods of prolonged vomiting. The nurse is observing the patient for signs of:
    1. metabolic acidosis.
    2. metabolic alkalosis.
    3. respiratory acidosis.
    4. respiratory alkalosis.

50. The nurse is working with a patient who has had emphysema for many years. The nurse believes that the patient has uncompensated respiratory acidosis. This belief is a result of an analysis of the patient's blood gas values that reveals:
    1. pH = 7.35, $Paco_2$ = 40 mm Hg, HCO_3^- concentration = 22 mEq/L.
    2. pH = 7.40, $Paco_2$ = 45 mm Hg, HCO_3^- concentration = 28 mEq/L.
    3. pH = 7.30, $Paco_2$ = 50 mm Hg, HCO_3^- concentration = 24 mEq/L.
    4. pH = 7.45, $Paco_2$ = 55 mm Hg, HCO_3^- concentration = 18 mEq/L.

51. The patient has been admitted to the medical center for stabilization of congestive heart failure. The physician has prescribed Lasix (a diuretic) for the patient. This patient should be observed for:
    1. diarrhea.
    2. edema.
    3. dysrhythmia.
    4. hyperactive reflexes.

52. The patient has a potassium level above the normal value. The nurse anticipates that treatment for this patient with hyperkalemia will include:
    1. fluid restrictions.
    2. foods high in potassium.
    3. administration of diuretics.
    4. IV infusion of calcium.

53. The patient has lost a large amount of body fluid. In assessment of this patient with hypovolemia (ECV deficit), the nurse expects to find:
    1. oliguria.
    2. hypertension.
    3. periorbital edema.
    4. neck vein distention.

54. The nurse is determining the care that is to be provided to the patients on the medical unit. There are a number of patients who have the potential for a fluid and electrolyte imbalance. A nurse-initiated (independent) intervention for these patients is:
    1. administration of IV fluids.
    2. monitoring of intake and output.
    3. performance of diagnostic tests.
    4. dietary replacement of necessary fluids/electrolytes.

55. For a patient who is experiencing an ECV excess, the nurse plans to determine the fluid status. The best way for the nurse to determine the fluid balance for the patient is to:
    1. obtain diagnostic test results.
    2. monitor IV fluid intake.
    3. weigh the patient daily.
    4. assess vital signs.

Copyright © 2019, Elsevier Inc. All Rights Reserved.

56. The patient is admitted to the trauma unit following an accident while using power tools at home. The patient experienced significant blood loss and required a large infusion of citrated blood. The nurse assesses this patient for the development of:
    1. urinary retention.
    2. poor skin turgor.
    3. increased blood pressure reading.
    4. positive Chvostek's sign.

57. The patient is experiencing a severe anxiety reaction and the respiratory rate has increased significantly. Nursing intervention for this patient who may develop respiratory alkalosis is:
    1. placing the patient in a sitting position.
    2. providing the patient with nasal oxygen.
    3. having the patient breathe into a paper bag.
    4. asking the patient to cough and deep breathe.

58. A patient with normal renal function is to be maintained NPO. An IV of 1000 mL of D_5W is ordered to infuse over 8 hours. The nurse should:
    1. infuse the IV at a faster rate.
    2. add multivitamins to the solution.
    3. provide oral fluids as a supplement.
    4. question the prescriber about adding potassium to the IV.

59. A patient with an IV infusion may develop phlebitis. The nurse recognizes this condition by the presence at the IV infusion site of:
    1. pallor.
    2. swelling.
    3. redness.
    4. cyanosis.

60. The patient has had an IV line inserted. Upon observation of the IV site, the nurse notes that there is evidence of an infiltration. The nurse should first:
    1. slow the infusion.
    2. discontinue the infusion.
    3. change the IV bag and tubing.
    4. contact the prescriber immediately.

61. The nurse is reviewing the hospital policy for maintenance of IV infusions. The current guidelines for changing continuous IV tubing (non–blood administration sets) are every:
    1. 36 hours.
    2. 48 hours.
    3. 72 hours.
    4. 96 hours.

62. The patient has just started to receive the blood transfusion. The nurse is performing the patient assessment and notes the patient has chills and flank pain. The nurse stops the infusion and then:
    1. calls the physician.
    2. administers epinephrine.
    3. collects a urine specimen.
    4. sets up new tubing with an IV infusion of 0.9% saline.

63. A patient who has been admitted with a renal dysfunction is demonstrating signs and symptoms of an ECV excess (hypervolemia). Upon completing the patient assessment, the nurse anticipates finding:
    1. poor skin turgor.
    2. weight loss.
    3. increased blood pressure.
    4. increased urine specific gravity.

64. The nurse is assisting the patient with a fluid volume deficit to select an optimum replacement fluid. The nurse suggests that the patient drink:
    1. tea.
    2. milk.
    3. coffee.
    4. fruit juice.

65. A patient with congestive heart failure and fluid retention is placed on a fluid restriction of 1000 mL/24 hours. On the basis of guidelines for patients with restrictions, for the time period from 7:00 A.M. to 3:30 P.M. the nurse plans to provide the patient:
    1. 250 mL.
    2. 400 mL.
    3. 500 mL.
    4. 750 mL.

66. In accordance with the Infusion Nurses Society, a phlebitis grade of 2 is indicated for which of the following assessments?
    1. Erythema at access site with or without pain
    2. Pain at access site with erythema and/or edema
    3. Pain at access site with erythema, streak formation, palpable venous cord
    4. Pain at access site with erythema, streak formation, palpable venous cord >2.5 cm (1 inch) in length, purulent drainage

67. The patient has a history of alcoholism and is admitted to the medical center in a malnourished state. The nurse specifically checks the lab values for:
    1. hypercalcemia.
    2. hyponatremia.
    3. hyperkalemia.
    4. hypomagnesemia.

Copyright © 2019, Elsevier Inc. All Rights Reserved.

68. The patient who is most prone to respiratory acidosis is the individual who is experiencing;
    1. hyperthyroidism.
    2. an acute asthma episode.
    3. renal failure.
    4. an anxiety reaction.

69. Older adults have a greater risk of fluid imbalance as a result of;
    1. increased thirst response.
    2. decreased glomerular filtration.
    3. increased body fluid percentage.
    4. increased basal metabolic rate.

70. An example of a type of medication that can lead to metabolic acidosis is:
    1. penicillin.
    2. aldactone.
    3. potassium.
    4. Benadryl.

71. An appropriate technique when initiating an intravenous infusion is to:
    1. use hard, stiff veins.
    2. shave the arm hair with a razor.
    3. use the proximal site in the dominant arm.
    4. apply the tourniquet 4–6 inches above the selected site.

72. A unit of packed cells or whole blood usually transfuses over:
    1. ½ hour.
    2. 1 hour.
    3. 2 hours.
    4. 5 hours.

73. An individual with type O blood is able to receive:
    1. type A or type B.
    2. type AB.
    3. type O.
    4. all types.

74. A specific technique for initiating intravenous therapy for an older adult is to:
    1. select sites in the hands.
    2. use the largest possible IV cannula gauge.
    3. set the IV flow rate at 150–200 mL/hour.
    4. insert at a decreased angle of 10–15 degrees.

75. The patient lost 4 pounds since last week as a result of taking Lasix. This is approximately:
    1. ½ L of fluid.
    2. 1 L of fluid.
    3. 2 L of fluid.
    4. 4 L of fluid.

76. The patient has respiratory alkalosis. The nurse expects to assess which of the following signs?
    1. Decreased respirations
    2. Muscle twitching
    3. Abdominal distention
    4. Hyperactive reflexes

77. For patients receiving anticoagulants, the nurse should apply pressure after the removal of the IV for at least:
    1. 1 minute.
    2. 2 minutes.
    3. 5 minutes.
    4. 20 minutes.

78. The nurse is troubleshooting that is infusing too slowly. What action is indicated first?
    1. Remove the IV from the site.
    2. Check the IV catheter for kinking or dislodgement.
    3. Increase the rate of the infusion.
    4. Change the IV fluid bag and tubing.

STUDY GROUP QUESTIONS

- How are body fluids distributed in the body?
- What is the composition of body fluids?
- How do fluids move throughout the body?
- How is the intake of body fluids regulated?
- What are the major electrolytes, and what is their function in the body?
- How is acid-base balance maintained?
- What are the major fluid, electrolyte, and acid-base imbalances and their causes?
- What signs and symptoms will the patient exhibit in the presence of a fluid, electrolyte, or acid-base imbalance?
- What diagnostic tests are used to determine the presence of imbalances?
- What information is critical to obtain in a patient assessment in order to determine the presence of a fluid, electrolyte, or acid-base imbalance?
- What health deviations increase a patient's susceptibility to an imbalance?
- What nursing interventions should be implemented for patients with various fluid, electrolyte, and acid-base imbalances?
- What information should be included in patient/family teaching for prevention of imbalances, or restoration of fluid, electrolyte, or acid-base balance?
- What are the nursing responsibilities associated with the initiation and maintenance of IV therapy?
- What are the responsibilities of the nurse with regard to blood transfusions?

Copyright © 2019, Elsevier Inc. All Rights Reserved.

a. *Create study charts to compare:*
   i. *Electrolyte Imbalances and Patient Responses,* including etiology, diagnostic test results, patient assessment, and nursing interventions for sodium, potassium, calcium, and magnesium imbalances.
   ii. *Acid-Base Imbalances and Patient Responses,* including etiology, diagnostic test results, patient assessment, and nursing interventions both for metabolic acidosis and alkalosis and for respiratory acidosis and alkalosis.

   iii. *ECV Deficit and Excess and Patient Responses,* including etiology, diagnostic test results, patient assessment, and nursing interventions for both fluid excess and deficit.

b. Examine how the QSEN competency for safety is implemented for patients with intravenous infusions.

Copyright © 2019, Elsevier Inc. All Rights Reserved.

19 Complementary, Alternative, and Integrative Therapies

PRELIMINARY READING

Chapter 19, pp. 536–550

CASE STUDIES

1. You make a home visit to a patient who has painful osteoarthritis. The patient tells you that she has some herbal remedies on hand that she believes are more effective than the analgesic that has been ordered by the physician.
   a. What is your initial intervention after the patient has told you this information?

2. The patient is a military veteran who has episodes of PTSD. He does not want to take medication, if it can be avoided.
   a. What therapy would you recommend that the patient could investigate?

CHAPTER REVIEW

Match the description/definition in Column A with the correct term in Column B.

Column A	Column B
_____ 1. Burning a cone or stick of dried herbs that has healing properties on or near the skin	a. Tai chi
_____ 2. Represent opposing yet complementary phenomena that exist in a state of dynamic equilibrium	b. Integrative nursing
_____ 3. Conventional Western medicine	c. Qi gong
_____ 4. Mind-body technique that uses instruments to teach self-regulation and voluntary self-control over specific physiological responses	d. Complementary therapy
_____ 5. Originally a martial art that is now viewed as a moving meditation in which patients move their bodies slowly, gently, and with awareness while breathing deeply	e. Acupuncture
	f. Imagery
_____ 6. Conventional and complementary approaches are brought together in a coordinated way	g. Allopathic
_____ 7. Originally a martial art, now viewed as a series of carefully choreographed movements or gestures designed to promote the flow of energy in the body	h. Biofeedback
	i. Moxibustion
_____ 8. When a non-mainstream practice is used together with conventional medicine	j. Yin and yang
_____ 9. Mind-body therapy that uses the conscious mind for visualization to stimulate physical changes in the body, improve perceived well-being, and/or enhance self-awareness	
_____ 10. Regulates or realigns the vital energy, which flows like a river through the body in channels that form a system of 20 pathways called meridians	

Copyright © 2019, Elsevier Inc. All Rights Reserved.

Complete the following:

11. Identify at least five types of complementary therapies.

12. Historically, nurses have practiced in an integrative fashion.

    True _____   False _____

13. What are the five considerations when recommending complementary and integrative health approaches?

14. Indicate which of the following occur during the relaxation response. Select all that apply.

    a. Increased heart rate _____

    b. Decreased alpha brain activity _____

    c. Decreased blood pressure _____

    d. Increased neural impulses to the brain _____

    e. Increased peripheral skin temperature _____

    f. Decreased respiratory rate _____

15. Progressive relaxation should be done in a _____ order.

16. Identify at least four benefits of relaxation therapy.

17. Florence Nightingale practiced animal-companion therapy for her sick and disabled patients.

    True _____   False _____

18. What are the four methods that are used in Traditional Chinese Medicine (TCM) to evaluate a patient's condition?

19. People's use of herbal remedies is a new practice.

    True _____   False _____

20. The patient goes to the outpatient center on a weekly basis for chemotherapy. While having the chemotherapy, the art therapist comes around and asks if the patient would like to participate in drawing. This therapy is being used as:

    Alternative _____   Complementary _____

21. Which of the following are considered biofield therapies? Select all that apply.

    a. Reiki _____

    b. Accupressure _____

    c. Therapeutic touch _____

    d. Breathwork _____

    e. Yoga _____

22. An example of movement therapy is:

23. According to Traditional Chinese Medicine, what are the three causes of disease? Provide an example of each cause.

24. It is important to know which herbs to warn patients about using. Which of the following are identified as unsafe herbs? Select all that apply.

    a. Chaparral _____

    b. Black cohosh _____

    c. Life root _____

    d. Licorice _____

    e. Coltsfoot _____

    f. Aloe _____

25. For an older adult, to prevent "skin hunger" the nurse needs to use:

26. Therapeutic touch is contraindicated for a patient who has:

27. Indicate the correct sequence for teaching a patient the *4-7-8* breath.

    a. Hold your breath for a count of seven. _____

    b. Exhale completely through your mouth, making a whoosh sound to a count of eight. _____

    c. This is one breath. Now inhale again and repeat the cycle three more times for a total of four breaths. _____

    d. Exhale completely through your mouth, making a "whoosh" sound. _____

    e. Close your mouth and inhale quietly through your nose to a mental count of four. _____

Copyright © 2019, Elsevier Inc. All Rights Reserved.

28. Complementary therapies require commitment and regular involvement by a patient to be most effective and have prolonged beneficial outcomes.

True _____   False _____

Select the best answer for each of the following questions:

29. The patient tells you that she uses an herbal product for upper respiratory tract infections. You anticipate that the product used is:
    1. feverfew.
    2. echinacea.
    3. ginseng.
    4. saw palmetto.

30. A patient has been taking valerian to assist with sleeping and mild anxiety. Because of its effect, you will monitor for possible interaction with:
    1. barbiturates.
    2. anticoagulants.
    3. loop diuretics.
    4. corticosteroids.

31. The nurse is preparing a presentation on alternative therapies for a community group. The nurse should indicate that herbal therapies are:
    1. approved by the Food and Drug Administration, under the Food, Drug, and Cosmetic Act.
    2. sold as medicines in most stores because they lack major side effects.
    3. allowed to be packaged as dietary supplements if they are without health claims.
    4. consistent in their standards for concentrations of major ingredients and additives.

32. The patient asks the nurse about different herbal therapies that may promote physical endurance and improve immune function. Based on the patient's request, the nurse provides information on:
    1. ginseng.
    2. ginger.
    3. echinacea.
    4. chamomile.

33. The nurse is aware of the positive responses that may be obtained with the use of alternative therapies. A benefit that the patient can gain from relaxation therapy is a decrease in:
    a. receptivity.
    b. peripheral skin temperature.
    c. oxygen consumption.
    d. alpha brain activity.

34. In selecting an appropriate alternative therapy, the nurse knows that the patient who may benefit the most from the passive type of relaxation is one who is experiencing:
    1. hypertension.
    2. terminal cancer.
    3. work-related stress.
    4. dysfunctional grieving.

35. A nurse needs to be alert to possible negative responses to biobehavioral therapies. Patients who have reacted negatively have most often experienced:
    1. aggressive behaviors.
    2. delusions.
    3. insomnia.
    4. loss of control sensations.

36. A practitioner or patient who uses Traditional Chinese Medicine bases the therapy upon the primary concept of:
    1. yin and yang.
    2. meridians.
    3. six senses.
    4. acupoints.

37. The patient has a history of gastrointestinal problems and has used herbal remedies in the past. The nurse expects that this patient has taken:
    1. chamomile.
    2. St. John's wort.
    3. echinacea.
    4. gingko biloba.

38. A patient at the clinic informs the nurse during an examination that he has been taking comfrey as an antiinflammatory for osteoarthritis. The patient asks if there is any reason this remedy should not be taken. The nurse responds accurately when telling the patient that chaparral:
    1. may induce kidney disease.
    2. should not be taken with coffee or other caffeinated beverages.
    3. is associated with liver toxicity and venoocclusive disease.
    4. is unsafe for people with diabetes.

39. In selecting an appropriate alternative therapy, the nurse knows that the pediatric patient who has chronic pain may benefit the most from:
    1. relaxation therapy.
    2. imagery.
    3. biofeedback.
    4. acupuncture.

40. Which of the following patients is not a good candidate for animal-companion therapy?
    1. A child with ADHD
    2. An adult with MRSA
    3. A lonely adult
    4. An adult with depression

Copyright © 2019, Elsevier Inc. All Rights Reserved.

STUDY GROUP QUESTIONS

- What are complementary, alternative, and integrative therapies?
- How should patients be assessed for the use of CAM?
- What are the benefits and limitations of complementary and alternative therapies?
- Which patients will benefit the most from specific therapies?
- What are the contraindications for specific therapies?
- Which types of therapies are nurse accessible and which are training specific?
- Which disorders may benefit from herbal remedies?
- Which herbal remedies interact with prescription medications?
- How are herbal remedies safely distributed?
- Which herbs are unsafe to use?

Copyright © 2019, Elsevier Inc. All Rights Reserved.

20 Caring in Nursing Practice

PRELIMINARY READING

Chapter 20, pp. 551–562

CASE STUDIES

1. The daughter of a patient in an extended care facility has traveled from another state to visit. When she arrives with her husband and teenage son, she finds that her mother has deteriorated dramatically from the last time she spoke with her. The patient, in the terminal stages of liver disease, is now only minimally responsive with episodes of agitation and disorientation. The family, especially the daughter, is emotionally distraught.
   a. What can be done by the nurse to demonstrate caring for this patient's family?
   b. What can be done for the patient to demonstrate caring?

2. The nurse observes the student giving a bath to a bedridden patient. The door to the room is open and the patient is exposed. In addition, the student is not being very gentle with the patient.
   a. What caring behaviors are missing?
   b. How can the nurse help the student to recognize and incorporate caring behaviors?

CHAPTER REVIEW

Complete the following:

1. Match the theorists with the theoretical concepts:
   Patricia Benner and Judith Wrubel
   Jean Watson
   Madeleine Leininger
   Kristen Swanson

   a. Five processes and subdimensions _____

   b. Transpersonal caring _____

   c. Caring is primary _____

   d. Transcultural caring _____

2. For the following nursing behaviors, identify a specfic example of a clinical intervention.
   a. Providing presence
   b. Comforting/touch
   c. Listening
   d. Knowing the patient

3. A patient is to have an IV line inserted. The nurse demonstrates caring behaviors by:

4. Describe how caring and spirituality are connected.

5. How can nurses care for each other?

6. Identify three actions that are perceived by a patient's family as the nurse demonstrating caring.

Select the best answer for each of the following questions:

7. A nurse is discussing with her peers how much a patient matters to her. She states that she does not want the patient to suffer. The nurse is implementing the theory described by:
   1. Patricia Benner.
   2. Jean Watson.
   3. Kristen Swanson.
   4. Madeleine Leininger.

8. A patient was admitted to the hospital to have diagnostic tests to rule out a cancerous lesion in the lungs. The nurse is sitting with the patient in the room awaiting the results of the tests. The nurse is demonstrating the caring behavior of:
   1. knowing.
   2. comforting.
   3. providing presence.
   4. maintaining belief.

9. A nurse manager would like to promote more opportunities for the staff on the busy unit to demonstrate caring behaviors. The manager elects to implement:
   1. more time off for the staff.
   2. a strict schedule for patient treatments.
   3. staff input into patient assignments.
   4. hospital committee appointments.

Copyright © 2019, Elsevier Inc. All Rights Reserved.

10. A new graduate is looking at theories of caring. He selects Leininger's theory because it is most agreeable with his belief system. Leininger defines caring as a(n):
1. new consciousness and moral idea.
2. nurturing way of relating to a valued other.
3. central, unifying domain necessary for health and survival.
4. improvement in the human condition using a transcultural perspective.

11. A nurse is working with a patient who has been admitted to the oncology unit for treatment of a cancerous growth. This nurse is applying Swanson's theory of caring and demonstrating the concept of maintaining belief when:
1. performing the patient's dressing changes.
2. providing explanations about the medications.
3. keeping the patient draped during the physical exam.
4. discussing how the radiation therapy will assist in decreasing the tumor's size.

12. A new graduate is assigned to a surgical unit where there are a large number of procedures to be performed during each shift. This nurse demonstrates a caring behavior in this situation by:
1. avoiding situations that may be uncomfortable or difficult.
2. attempting to do all the treatments independently and quickly.
3. seeking assistance before performing new or difficult skills.
4. telling patients that he or she is a new graduate and unfamiliar with all the procedures.

13. An example of the caring process of "enabling" is:
1. performing a catheter insertion quickly and well.
2. reassuring the patient that the lab results should be fine.
3. providing pain medication before a procedure.
4. assisting a patient during the birth of a child.

14. A subdimension of Swanson's process of caring— "doing for others as he/she would do for self"— involves:
1. being there.
2. performing skillfully.
3. generating alternatives.
4. offering realistic optimism.

15. In the Caring Assessment Tool (CAT), an example of mutual problem solving with a patient is when a nurse:
1. discusses health issues with the patient and family.
2. pays attention to the patient.
3. provides privacy for the patient.
4. includes the family members in the patient's care.

16. A nurse attempts to understand the specific cultural concerns of a patient and how they relate to his illness. What caring factor is applied?
1. Attentive reassurance
2. Encouragement
3. Provision of basic human needs
4. Appreciation of unique meanings

17. Additional teaching is required if a nurse observes a nursing assistant working with an older adult patient and:
1. has the patient select the clothes to wear.
2. addresses the patient as "Honey."
3. carefully organizes the patient's personal items.
4. combs and styles the patient's hair.

18. In a caring environment, the nurse specifically meets the patient's affiliation needs by:
1. being responsive to the family.
2. accepting his/her personal beliefs.
3. helping with routine needs.
4. being interested in his/her concerns.

STUDY GROUP QUESTIONS

- What is "caring" in the nursing profession?
- What are the major theories of caring and the key concepts in each one?
- How is caring perceived by patients?
- What are caring behaviors?
- How can a nurse demonstrate caring to patients and families?

Copyright © 2019, Elsevier Inc. All Rights Reserved.

21 Cultural Competence

PRELIMINARY READING

Chapter 21, pp. 563–577

CASE STUDY

1. For the following situations, identify how a nurse should approach the patient and significant others in order to recognize cultural concerns and health care needs:
   a. Large numbers of family members surround the patient on the acute care unit.
   b. Dietary practices of the patient prohibit the eating of meat or meat products.
   c. A traditional healer makes calls to the patient's home between the patient's visits to the physician.
   d. The patient and her family speak another language.

CHAPTER REVIEW

Match the description/definition in Column A with the correct term in Column B.

Column A

_____ 1. Determines how people perceive others, how they interact and relate to reality, and how they process information

_____ 2. "A particular type of health difference that is closely linked with social, economic, and/or environmental disadvantage"

_____ 3. Key quality indicators that help health care institutions improve performance, increase accountability, and reduce costs

_____ 4. A research and policy model used to study the complexities of people's lives and experiences

_____ 5. The conditions in which persons are born, grow, live, work, and age

_____ 6. People who are gay, lesbian, bisexual, or transgender; people of color; people who are physically and/or mentally challenged; and people who are not college educated

_____ 7. An ongoing process in which a health care professional tries to achieve the ability and availability to effectively work within the cultural context of a patient

_____ 8. When care fits a person's life patterns, values, and system of meaning

Column B

a. Marginalized groups

b. Cultural competence

c. Core measures

d. Health disparity

e. Intersectionality

f. Social determinants of health

g. World view

h. Culturally congruent care

Complete the following:

9. Provide an example for how the nurse may develop each of the following.
   a. Cultural awareness

   b. Cultural skills

10. Identify an example of a question a nurse could use to elicit specific cultural information from a patient regarding health beliefs and practices.

11. Identify the benefit of transcultural communication.

12. Explain linguistic competence.

92

Copyright © 2019, Elsevier Inc. All Rights Reserved.

13. Identify two examples of marginalized groups and their health care challenges.

14. What should be incorporated into "teach-back" to address cultural considerations?

15. Identify four important aspects for working with an interpreter.

16. What are the parts of the LEARN mnemonic?
    L:
    E:
    A:
    R:
    N:

17. Identify at least 3 of the 12 domains of culture.

18. In 2011, 30.3% or approximately 84 million persons in the United States did not have at least one healthier food retailer within the census tract or within ½ mile of tract boundaries.

    True _____   False _____

19. Provide an example of how storytelling can be used to understand a patient's cultural perspective.

Select the best answer for each of the following questions:

20. A nurse is meeting a patient for the first time for the admission interview. There are eight family members sitting around the patient's bed. After introductions, the most appropriate nursing action is to:
    1. come back at another time.
    2. proceed with the admission interview.
    3. ask the family members to leave immediately.
    4. ask the patient if he or she wants a family member present.

21. The community center where a nurse volunteers has a culturally diverse population. The nurse wants to promote communication with all the patients from different cultures. A beneficial technique for the nurse is to:
    1. explain nursing terms that are used.
    2. use constant eye contact and touch with all patients.
    3. call patients by their first names to establish rapport.
    4. expect responses to all questions that are asked.

22. When working with an interpreter for a patient who speaks another language, the nurse should:
    1. direct questions to the interpreter.
    2. expect word-for-word translation.
    3. ensure that the interpreter speaks the patient's dialect.
    4. ask the interpreter to evaluate the patient's non-verbal behaviors.

23. Which of the following questions is appropriate to use to determine the patient's parenting style/family roles?
    1. Are there particular methods being used for treatment of illness?
    2. Who makes the decisions in the family?
    3. Is there a religion or faith to which the patient adheres?
    4. Is touch an acceptable form of communication?

STUDY GROUP QUESTIONS

- What is culture?
- What are some of the marginalized groups in the country/community and their health challenges?
- How can a nurse promote communication with individuals who are from other cultures and/or individuals who speak different languages?
- How can a nurse identify and respond to a patient's cultural needs?
- What information may be obtained from a cultural assessment?
- What nursing approaches may be successful in assisting multicultural patients in health care settings?
- What resources are available to assist a nurse in learning about and working with patients from other cultures?

Copyright © 2019, Elsevier Inc. All Rights Reserved.

22 Spiritual Health

PRELIMINARY READING

Chapter 22, pp. 578–596

CASE STUDY

1. A nurse is working in an acute care facility with a patient who practices Buddhism.
   a. What information should be obtained in relation to the patient's spiritual practices?
   b. What adaptations may need to be made by the nurse, the other members of the health care team, and the acute care facility to meet the patient's spiritual needs?

CHAPTER REVIEW

Match the description/definition in Column A with the correct term in Column B.

Column A

_____ 1. Does not believe in the existence of a supreme spiritual being or god

_____ 2. Cultural or institutional religion; relationship with a divinity, higher power, authority, or spirit

_____ 3. Awareness of one's inner self and a sense of connection to a higher being

_____ 4. Multidimensional concept that gives comfort while a person endures hardship and challenges

_____ 5. Awareness of that which cannot be seen or known in ordinary ways

_____ 6. Belief that ultimate reality is unknown or unknowable

_____ 7. A dimension of spirituality that is related to the human need of belonging

Column B

a. Faith

b. Hope

c. Connectedness

d. Atheist

e. Spirituality

f. Self-transcendence

g. Agnostic

Complete the following:

8. Identify general nursing interventions for promotion of spiritual health.

9. An example of a nursing intervention for a patient who has had a near-death experience is:

10. Identify two possible patient outcomes relating to spirituality or spiritual health.

11. Identify what each letter in the FICA assessment tool acronym designates:
    F:
    I:
    C:
    A:

12. Formulate a question that may be asked to determine a patient's spiritual belief system.

13. There is an order for whole blood replacement for a patient. Before the blood administration, a nurse will check to see if the patient is a member of what religion(s)?

14. Provide at least two examples of rituals or practices associated with spirituality or religion.

Copyright © 2019, Elsevier Inc. All Rights Reserved.

15. Religious or spiritual practices may have an impact upon the provision of healthcare to a patient. For an individual who is of the Islamic faith, which of the following may need to be considered by a nurse and other health care providers? Select all that apply.

a. Organ donation will be approved. _____

b. Women prefer female providers/examiners. _____

c. Euthanasia is practiced. _____

d. Time will need to be set aside during the day for prayer. _____

e. Faith healing may be used. _____

f. Blood products and medicines may be refused. _____

16. Identify the four dimensions of spiritual well-being.

17. Indicate which of the following statements about spirituality is/are correct. Select all that apply.
a. Patients who identify a religious belief will all practice similar rituals. _____

b. Promoting spirituality can help a patient cope with illness. _____

c. Promoting a patient's spirituality may reduce the incidence of depression. _____

d. The link between spirituality and physical health is well understood. _____

e. Spirituality exists in all people regardless of their religious beliefs. _____

18. How does the nurse use presence to promote spiritual well-being?

19. The nurse wants to assist patients to achieve spiritual health. The nurse should:
(Select all that apply.)

a. solve their spiritual problems. _____

b. employ his/her own personal religious practices with the patient. _____

c. explore meditation with the patient to assist in reducing stress. _____

d. integrate patient preferences into the plan of care. _____

e. provide an environment for expression of beliefs. _____

f. recognize that all patients experience spiritual problems. _____

20. Patients who are not practicing a specific religion do not have spiritual needs.

True _____   False _____

Select the best answer for each of the following questions:

21. A patient is admitted to a medical center for surgery to repair a fractured hip. Upon reviewing the patient's admission history, a nurse finds that the patient attends religious services routinely. The nurse supports the patient's needs by stating:
1. "Do you really go to services often?"
2. "Don't worry. God will take care of you."
3. "I'll call your minister and have him stop by to see you."
4. "Is there any way that I may be able to help you with your spiritual needs?"

22. A patient who is of the Jewish faith is admitted to the long-term care facility. A nurse seeks to provide support of the usual health practices that are part of this religion. The nurse learns that one component of usual Jewish tradition states that:
1. no euthanasia should be used.
2. a faith healer will be involved.
3. modern medical treatment should be refused.
4. physical exams should be performed only by individuals of the same sex.

23. While caring for a patient in the intensive care unit, the patient has a cardiac arrest. The patient is successfully resuscitated. After this near-death experience, the patient is progressing physically, but appears withdrawn and concerned. The nurse assists the patient by stating:
1. "The experience that you had is easy to explain and understand."
2. "That was a very close call. It must be very frightening for you."
3. "Other people have had similar experiences and worked through their feelings."
4. "If you would like to talk about your experience, I will stay with you."

Copyright © 2019, Elsevier Inc. All Rights Reserved.

24. For a patient with a diagnosis of a chronic disease, a nurse wishes to encourage feelings of hope. The nurse recognizes that hope provides a(n):
    1. meaning and purpose for the patient.
    2. organized approach to dealing with the disease process.
    3. connection to the cultural background of the patient.
    4. binding relationship with the divine being of the patient's religion.

25. A nurse is reviewing the plan of care for a 66-year-old home-care patient who is experiencing the beginning stages of Alzheimer disease. The nurse believes that the patient may need to be assessed for spiritual needs based on discovering:
    1. memory problems.
    2. a difficulty with ADLs.
    3. an inability to cope with the illness.
    4. a family history of the disease.

26. According to Erikson's stages of psychosocial development, with regard to spiritual beliefs it is expected that a 6-year-old child will:
    1. begin to ask about a god or supreme being.
    2. have spiritual well-being provided by the parents.
    3. interpret meanings literally.
    4. begin to learn the difference between right and wrong.

27. According to Erikson's stages of psychosocial development, with regard to spiritual beliefs it is expected that a middle-aged person will begin to:
    1. reflect on inconsistencies in religious stories.
    2. form independent beliefs and attitudes.
    3. review value systems during a crisis.
    4. sort fantasy from fact.

28. A young adult is diagnosed with a very aggressive form of cancer. He yells at the nurse, "Why did this happen to me?" The nurse's best response is:
    1. "Do you think that you did something wrong?"
    2. "You sound upset about your situation. Let's talk about it."
    3. "Tell me why you think this is unfair."
    4. "What makes you say that?"

29. The patient's family wants to bring in food that is approved for their religion. Which of the following is the best response by the nurse?
    1. "The patient cannot have foods that are brought in from outside of the hospital."
    2. "That would be great. Bring in anything that the patient likes to eat."
    3. "The most important thing is to make sure that everything is cooked well."
    4. "What type of food are you going to bring? Let's make sure that it fits with the prescribed diet."

30. The patient is told by a family member that it doesn't look like the treatments are working. What aspect of spiritual health is being threatened?
    1. Hope
    2. Vocation
    3. Connectedness
    4. Transcendence

STUDY GROUP QUESTIONS

- What is spirituality and how does it relate to an individual's health status?
- What are the concepts of spirituality/spiritual health?
- What spiritual or religious problems may arise during patient care?
- How can a nurse assess a patient's spirituality/spiritual health?
- What is the role of a nurse in promoting spiritual health?
- How can a nurse avoid imposing his or her own beliefs on a patient?
- What are the differences and similarities in spiritual practices and health beliefs among the major religious sects?
- How is hope related to spirituality?

Copyright © 2019, Elsevier Inc. All Rights Reserved.

23 Growth and Development

PRELIMINARY READING

Chapter 23, pp. 597–623

CASE STUDIES

1. A student nurse with an inpatient pediatric unit in a medical center has three patients—an infant, a 5-year-old child, and a 16-year-old adolescent.
   a. How should the nurse promote growth and developmental needs for these patients in the acute care environment?
   b. What would be included in a teaching plan for the new parents of the infant?

2. A patient in the extended care facility is an 86-year-old woman who is occasionally disoriented to time, place, and person.
   a. How should a nurse approach this patient to assist her in meeting her developmental needs?

3. A student nurse is working as a summer camp nurse with children 8 to 10 years old. It is the nurse's turn to select diversional activities for a group.
   a. What types of games or activities are appropriate for this age group?

4. A nurse is teaching the parents of adolescents the signs that may indicate a potential suicidal tendency in their children.
   a. What signs/behaviors will the nurse identify for these parents?
   b. What should be done if the individual is assessed as at risk for committing suicide?

5. The parents of an infant say that they are afraid to have their child vaccinated because they have "heard so many bad things about it."
   a. What can you explain to these parents regarding vaccinations and the benefits of having their child vaccinated??

CHAPTER REVIEW

Match the description in Column A with the correct theorist in Column B.

	Column A	*Column B*
_____	1. Development of cognition	a. Freud
_____	2. Psychosexual focus	b. Erikson
_____	3. Based on human needs	c. Maslow
_____	4. Moral development	d. Piaget
_____	5. Psychosocial development	e. Kohlberg

Complete the following:

6. a. An example of a teratogen is:

   b. Why are teratogens able to have an impact upon fetal development?

7. The leading cause of death in the toddler and pre-school age groups is:

Copyright © 2019, Elsevier Inc. All Rights Reserved.

8. Select the age group (infant, toddler, preschool age, school age, adolescent, young adult, middle-aged adult, or older adult) in which each of the following behaviors is evident or usually begins:
   a. Toilet training
   b. Tripling of birth weight
   c. Holding a pencil and printing letters
   d. Separation anxiety
   e. Moving away from the family
   f. Parallel play
   g. Search for personal identity
   h. Menopause
   i. Speaking in short sentences
   j. More graceful running and jumping
   k. Development of fears
   l. Decreased pitch discrimination
   m. Loss of primary teeth
   n. Development of primary and secondary sexual characteristics
   o. Low risk of chronic illness
   p. Diminished skin turgor and appearance of wrinkles
   q. Socioeconomic stability
   r. Recognition of objects by their outward appearance

9. To promote awareness of time, place, and person in an extended care environment, a nurse implements:

10. Prescriptive use or administration of more medication than indicated clinically is termed:

11. Identify safety concerns in the home environment for the following age groups:
    a. Toddler:
    b. Older adult:

12. What are the expected physical assessment findings for a middle-aged adult? Select all that apply.
    a. Abnormal visual fields and ocular movements _____
    b. Palpable lateral thyroid nodes _____
    c. Pulse rate of 60 to 100 beats per minute _____
    d. Decreased strength of abdominal muscles _____
    e. Responsive sensory system _____
    f. Diminished motor responses _____

13. Identify a topic area that is age-appropriate for a group of older adults in a senior housing development.

14. Indicate ways that the nurse can reduce stress for a hospitalized child.

15. a. Risk-taking behavior by the adolescent can lead to which health concerns?

    b. What is a potential nursing diagnosis for an adolescent individual?

16. What are the characteristics of the adolescent age group? Select all that apply.
    a. Preference for same sex peers _____
    b. Completion of language development _____
    c. Search for personal identify _____
    d. Following the rules of new authority figures _____
    e. Adoption of the parents' moral standards _____
    f. Development of secondary sex characteristics _____

17. How is the "Sandwich Generation" a challenge for nurses?

18. Identify at least one health concern for toddlers.

19. Indicate which of the following are true for older adult individuals. Select all that apply.
    a. Cognitive impairment is always expected. _____
    b. Strong visual memory is retained. _____
    c. Delirium is potentially reversible. _____
    d. Depression is becoming more common in this population. _____
    e. Short-term memory is unaffected. _____
    f. Sense of touch remains strong. _____

20. a. The single best predictor of adult hypertension is:

    b. The risk of hypertension is increased if the child is:

Copyright © 2019, Elsevier Inc. All Rights Reserved.

21. What are the concerns of internet and social media use for children and adolescents?

Select the best answer for each of the following questions:

22. A nurse is assigned to prepare a teaching plan for a group of preschool age children. For this age group, the nurse includes:
    1. appropriate use of medications.
    2. cooking safety including use of the stove.
    3. information on prevention of obesity and hypertension.
    4. guidelines for crossing the street or actions to take during a fire.

23. Children who are admitted to a hospital may be afraid about the hospitalization. To reduce the fear of school-age children in an acute care environment, a nurse:
    1. restrains them for all assessments and procedures.
    2. shows them the equipment that is to be used for procedures.
    3. provides in-depth information on how procedures are done.
    4. tells them that everything will be all right and the procedures will not hurt.

24. During a clinical rotation a student nurse is observing children in a day care center. The student is asked to assist with the activities for the preschool age children. Children in this age group are usually able to:
    1. make detailed drawings.
    2. classify objects by size or color.
    3. easily hold a pencil and print letters.
    4. use a vocabulary of more than 8000 words.

25. Parents of a toddler ask a nurse what their child should be able to do at the age of 2½ years old. The nurse identifies that the toddler will be able to:
    1. skip and throw a ball.
    2. speak in short sentences.
    3. solve difficult problems.
    4. recognize safety hazards.

26. Parents of a 1-year-old are asking about what can be expected of a child this age. A nurse informs the parents that a major milestone for a 1-year-old child is:
    1. tripling of the birth weight.
    2. sleeping 6–7 hours each day.
    3. walking with good balance.
    4. playing well with others.

27. A nurse is working with a group of young adults at the community center. There are many discussions about life and health issues. The nurse is aware that a health-related concern for young adults is that:
    1. attachment needs must be enhanced.
    2. "labeling" may alter their self-perceptions.
    3. adaptation to chronic disease is developing.
    4. fast-paced lifestyles may place them at risk for illnesses or disabilities.

28. A nurse is seeking to evaluate the effectiveness of information provided to the parents of an infant. The nurse determines that teaching has been successful when the parents:
    1. place small pillows in the infant's crib.
    2. position the infant on the stomach for sleeping.
    3. purchase a crib with slats that are less than 2 inches apart.
    4. prop up a bottle for the infant to suck on while falling asleep.

29. When presenting a program for a group of individuals in their middle-aged adult years, a nurse informs the members to expect the following physical change:
    1. a decrease in skin turgor.
    2. increased breast size.
    3. palpable lateral thyroid lobes.
    4. a visual acuity that is greater than 20/50.

30. An expected physical change for an older adult is:
    1. warmer extremities.
    2. increased perspiration.
    3. reduced adaptation to darkness.
    4. generalized erythema.

31. An adolescent girl has gone to a family-planning center for information about birth control. The patient asks the nurse what she should use to avoid getting pregnant. The nurse responds:
    1. "Are your parents aware of your sexual activity?"
    2. "You've been using some kind of protection before, right?"
    3. "What are your friends doing to protect themselves?"
    4. "What can you tell me about your past sexual experiences?"

32. A patient has gone to an outpatient obstetric clinic for a routine checkup. The patient asks a nurse what is happening with the baby now that she is in her second trimester. The nurse informs the patient that the:
    1. skin thickens and lanugo disappears.
    2. body becomes rounder and fuller.
    3. brain is undergoing a tremendous growth spurt.
    4. organ systems continue basic development and move toward refinement of function.

Copyright © 2019, Elsevier Inc. All Rights Reserved.

33. The nurse recognizes that there are changes that occur for the patient who has Alzheimer's disease. One of these is agnosia, which the nurse knows is the:
    1. loss of language skills.
    2. progressive loss of memory.
    3. loss of ability to recognize objects.
    4. loss of the ability to perform familiar tasks.

34. Which of the following is a potentially reversible cognitive impairment?
    1. Dementia
    2. Depression
    3. Disengagement
    4. Ischemic vascular dementia

STUDY GROUP QUESTIONS

- What are the principles of growth and development?
- How can growth and development be influenced?
- What are the differences and similarities of the major developmental theorists?

- How can a nurse apply the different developmental theories to patient situations?
- What are the major physical, psychosocial, and cognitive changes that occur throughout the life span?
- What are the specific health needs for each developmental stage?
- How does the approach of a nurse differ for individuals in each developmental stage to meet their developmental needs?
- What are the different teaching/learning needs of each developmental stage?

STUDY CHART

Create a study chart to compare *Growth and Development Across the Life Span* that identifies the physical abilities, psychosocial/cognitive activities, and health promotion behaviors and strategies for each age group from infancy to older adulthood.

Copyright © 2019, Elsevier Inc. All Rights Reserved.

24 Self-Concept and Sexuality

PRELIMINARY READING

Chapter 24, pp. 624–643

CASE STUDIES

1. A 22-year-old man is admitted to a rehabilitation facility. He was seriously injured in an automobile accident and now is paraplegic. Although medically stable, it appears that he is having difficulty dealing with his physical limitations. The patient speaks frequently about his girlfriend and his involvement in athletics and other social activities.
   a. What self-concept and sexuality issues are involved in this situation?
   b. Formulate a plan of care for this patient:

2. A nurse suspects that a patient is the victim of sexual abuse.
   a. What behaviors may the patient be exhibiting that would lead to this assessment?
   b. What questions should the nurse ask to get more information from the patient about the possible abuse?

3. Your patient has been on chemotherapy for 12 weeks. When you make a home visit, you observe that the patient appears fatigued, and he has lost a lot of hair and body weight. He tells you that he feels weak, feels bad about the loss of hair, which used to be darker and very thick, and he is upset that his wife has to do lifting, moving, and most of the household chores. Based upon this information:
   a. What are the self-concept issues that seem to be most important to this patient?
   b. What can you do to assist this patient to cope with these changes?

CHAPTER REVIEW

Match the description/definition in Column A with the correct term in Column B.

Column A	Column B
_____ 1. Set of conscious and unconscious feelings and beliefs about oneself	a. Sexuality
_____ 2. Set of behaviors that have been approved by family, community, and culture as appropriate in particular situations	b. Self-concept
_____ 3. Persons' identities in relation to the gender to which they are attracted	c. Transgender
_____ 4. Overall sense of personal worth or value	d. Self-esteem
_____ 5. Experiences and attitudes related to appearance and physical abilities	e. Sexual orientation
_____ 6. A person's thoughts and feeling about the body; a sense of femaleness or maleness	f. Role performance
_____ 7. People whose gender identity or expression is different than their sex at birth	g. Identity
_____ 8. The sense of individuality and being distinct and separate from others	h. Body image

Copyright © 2019, Elsevier Inc. All Rights Reserved.

Complete the following:

9. Identify at least two examples of the following:
   a. Positive influences on self-concept

   b. Stressors to self-concept

10. Which of the following behaviors may indicate an altered self-concept? Select all that apply.

    a. Eye contact maintained _____

    b. Straight posture _____

    c. Hesitant speech _____

    d. Overly angry response _____

    e. Independence _____

    f. Passive attitude _____

    g. Ability to make decisions _____

    h. Unkempt appearance _____

11. For the following patients, identify the potential concerns related to self-concept and sexuality:
    a. A woman who has had a mastectomy:

    b. A woman who is undergoing chemotherapy for cancer and who has a young child at home:

    c. A 7-year-old child who has been severely burned:

    d. A middle-aged adult man who has had a heart attack:

12. A way in which a nurse may promote self-concept in an acute care setting is by:

13. An example of an alteration in sexual health is:

14. Specify an area for patient education to promote sexual health.

15. For a patient with low self-esteem because of being unable to successfully pass a required college course, identify a patient goal/outcome and nursing interventions.

16. The capacity for sexuality diminishes significantly in older adults.

    True _____ False _____

17. Cultural background does not directly influence self-concept.

    True _____ False _____

18. The best method of birth control to reinforce with patients is the least expensive selection.

    True _____ False _____

19. An example of an intervention that a nurse may implement to promote self-concept for an older adult is:

20. Briefly define the following sexual orientations:
    a. Transgender

    b. Questioning

    c. Asexual or aromantic

    d. Fluid

21. Provide an example of a role performance stressor.

22. a. The vaccine that is recommended for early adolescent males and females to reduce the risk for HPV-related cancers is:

    b. What is the recommended age range for this vaccination?

    c. What is the best schedule for receipt of the vaccine?

23. What medical diagnoses can interfere with sexual functioning?

24. How can the media have an impact upon body image?

Copyright © 2019, Elsevier Inc. All Rights Reserved.

25. The nurse makes a disapproving facial expression when seeing a transgender patient.
   a. What affect can this have on the patient?

   b. What can be done by the nurse to prevent this?

26. The nurse is going to speak with a female patient about different contraceptive methods. Indicate which of the following are correct. Select all that apply.
   a. Have the discussion in the examination room before she dresses to leave. _____

   b. Plan so there are no interruptions. _____

   c. Consider your patient's cultural and religious beliefs. _____

   d. Review only the methods that are considered most reliable. _____

   e. Encourage use of the method that will be used most consistently. _____

27. Cyberbullying has become an issue with the increased use of social media, e-mail, chat rooms, texting, and instant messaging.
   a. What should you look for in an assessment to see if an individual may be a victim of cyberbullying?

   b. What interventions should be implemented if the individual has been victimized?

28. What is the PLISSIT Model for assessing and approaching sexuality?

Select the best answer for each of the following questions:

29. A nurse recognizes that which of the following age groups are most vulnerable to identity stressors?
   1. Infancy
   2. Preschool
   3. Adolescence
   4. Middle-aged adulthood

30. An adolescent has gone to the nurse's office in a school to discuss some personal issues. The nurse wishes to determine the sexual health of this adolescent. The nurse begins by asking:
   1. "Do you use contraception?"
   2. "Have you already had sexual relations?"
   3. "Are your parents aware of your sexual activity?"
   4. "Do you have any concerns about sex or your body's development?"

31. During an interview and physical assessment of a female patient in the clinic, a nurse finds that the patient has multiple lacerations and bruises and that she has experienced headaches and difficulty sleeping. The nurse suspects:
   1. sexual dysfunction.
   2. emotional conflict.
   3. sexually transmitted disease.
   4. physical and/or sexual abuse.

32. A patient is admitted to a coronary care unit after an acute myocardial infarction. He tells the nurse, "I won't be able to do what I used to at the hardware store." The nurse recognizes that the patient is experiencing a problem with the self-concept component of:
   1. role performance.
   2. identity.
   3. self-esteem.
   4. body image.

33. An adolescent patient has just been diagnosed with scoliosis and will need to wear a corrective brace. She tells the nurse angrily, "I don't know why I have to have this stupid problem!" The nurse responds most appropriately by saying:
   1. "Tell me what you do when you get angry and upset."
   2. "Don't be angry. You'll be getting the best care available."
   3. "You'll heal quickly and the brace can come off pretty soon."
   4. "It's okay to be angry around your friends, but try not to be upset around your parents."

34. During an initial assessment at an outpatient clinic, a nurse wants to determine a patient's perception of identity. The nurse asks the patient:
   1. "What is your usual day like?"
   2. "How would you describe yourself?"
   3. "What activities do you enjoy doing at home?"
   4. "What changes would you make in your personal appearance?"

35. A patient has been in the rehabilitation facility for several weeks after a cerebral vascular accident (CVA/stroke). During the hospitalization, a nurse has identified that the patient has become progressively more depressed about his physical condition. Although the patient is able, he will not participate in personal grooming and now is refusing any visitors. At this point, the nurse intervenes by:
   1. telling the patient to think more positively about the future.
   2. helping the patient to get washed and dressed every day.
   3. leaving the patient to complete activities of daily living independently.
   4. contacting the physician to discuss a psychological consultation.

Copyright © 2019, Elsevier Inc. All Rights Reserved.

36. A nurse is working with a patient who has had a colostomy. The patient asks about resuming a sexual relationship with a partner. The nurse begins by determining:
    1. the patient's knowledge about sexual activity.
    2. how the patient felt about life changes in the past.
    3. the partner's feelings about the colostomy.
    4. how comfortable the patient and the partner are in communicating with each other.

37. A nurse who is using Erikson's theory expects that a 5-year-old boy will begin to:
    1. accept body changes and maturation.
    2. incorporate feedback from peers into his personality.
    3. distinguish himself from the environment around him.
    4. identify with a specific gender group.

38. A patient asks a nurse about a prescription for tadalafil (Cialis). The nurse recognizes, however, that this drug is contraindicated for the patient who is taking:
    1. antibiotics.
    2. antihypertensives.
    3. antihistamines.
    4. nonsteroidal antiinflammatory agents.

39. A nurse is aware that which of the following strategies is appropriate for teaching a patient for promotion of a positive sexual experience?
    1. Encouraging the use of only one position for intercourse
    2. Instructing couples to work harder at the beginning of intercourse
    3. Discussing side effects of medications that may alter responsiveness
    4. Emphasizing a shorter period of foreplay

40. Correction is required if a new nurse in the women's clinic is observed:
    1. closing the door during an examination.
    2. determining the patient's cultural beliefs.
    3. identifying physiological changes for the patient.
    4. discussing findings with the patient in the waiting room.

41. Which of the following is anticipated as a sexual change related to the aging process?
    1. Increased vaginal secretions
    2. Decreased time for ejaculation to be achieved
    3. Decreased time for maintenance of an erection
    4. Increased orgasmic contractions

42. During an initial assessment at an outpatient clinic, a nurse wants to determine a patient's level of self-esteem. The nurse asks the patient:
    1. "What is your usual day like?"
    2. "How do you feel about yourself?"
    3. "What hobbies do you enjoy doing at home?"
    4. "What changes would you make in your personal appearance?"

43. Which of the following statements should be a concern to the nurse who is interviewing a patient after a lower leg amputation?
    1. "People have always told me that I am resourceful."
    2. "I can adjust to what I will have to do differently."
    3. "I'm going to have to figure out a different type of exercise program."
    4. "I don't think that my husband is going to think I'm attractive enough now."

STUDY GROUP QUESTIONS

- What are the components of self-concept?
- What stressors may influence an individual's self-concept?
- How can a nurse promote an individual's self-concept in different health care settings?
- What is sexuality and how does it develop throughout the life span?
- How can sexual health be defined?
- What are some of the current issues related to sexuality and sexual health?
- How may sexual health be altered?
- What health-related factors may influence sexual function?
- How are self-concept and sexuality related?
- How can a nurse determine an individual's self-concept and sexual health?
- What adaptations may be made by a nurse in approaching different age groups for the assessment and promotion of self-concept and sexual health?
- How can a nurse apply critical thinking and nursing processes to the areas of self-concept and sexuality?
- What resources are available to assist individuals to promote optimum self-concept and sexual health?
- How can a nurse make the patient feel more at ease when completing an assessment of sexual health?

STUDY CHART

Create a study chart on *Stressors Affecting Self-Concept* that identifies how the components of self-concept may be influenced and nursing interventions that may be implemented to promote a patient's positive self-concept.

Copyright © 2019, Elsevier Inc. All Rights Reserved.

25 Family Dynamics

PRELIMINARY READING

Chapter 25, pp. 644–662

CASE STUDIES

1. A 65-year-old man has been admitted to the coronary care unit in a medical center. The patient experienced a myocardial infarction (heart attack) while working late in his store. His wife, who accompanied him to the medical center, not only has been the "homemaker" for the family for more than 25 years but also has assisted in the family business run by her husband. They have two children who live on their own. Their son lives with his male partner, and their younger daughter is married and has two children of her own. The patient and his wife speak readily about their daughter, but avoid talking about their son.
   a. What factors related to family roles and function are involved in this situation?
   b. What stage of the family life cycle is this family in currently?
   c. What strategies may a nurse use to promote communication in this family?
   d. How may the role of the patient and his wife influence the health education plan?
   e. Identify a family-oriented nursing diagnosis for this situation.

2. The visiting nurse is working with a patient who has just been discharged from a rehabilitation facility following hip surgery.
   a. What should be included in the environmental assessment for this patient?
   b. What information about the patient's family should be assessed?

CHAPTER REVIEW

Match the family stages in Column A with the key principle identified for that stage in Column B.

Column A	Column B
_____ 1. Unattached young adult	a. Increasing flexibility of family's boundaries to include children's independence
_____ 2. Newly married couple	b. Accepting parent-offspring separation
_____ 3. Family with adolescents	c. Accepting shifting of generational roles
_____ 4. Family with young adults	d. Committing to a new system
_____ 5. Family in later life	e. Accepting a multitude of exits from and entries into the family system

Complete the following:

6. What is a family?

7. How can genetic factors have an influence upon a family?

8. Identify what is meant by the following:
   a. Family hardiness

b. Family resiliency

c. Family diversity

9. Identify the major concerns or challenges that may influence families today.

Copyright © 2019, Elsevier Inc. All Rights Reserved.

10. For families providing care for a family member:
    a. Identify possible indicators of caregiver stress.

    b. Identify a nursing diagnosis for a family coping with the difficult care of an older adult parent in the home.

11. Which of the following are correct statements regarding today's society? Select all that apply.
    a. Statistics show that approximately 20% of marriages will end in divorce. _____

    b. The number of people living alone is expanding. _____

    c. Approximately 75% of people 15 years of age and older are married. _____

    d. Mothers head about 85% of single-parent families. _____

    e. Approximately 40% of same-sex couples are married. _____

    f. The fastest growing age group is 65 years and older. _____

12. Identify an effect that inadequate functioning may have on a family.

13. What questions may be asked to determine the influence of culture on a family?

14. Provide examples of health promotion interventions for a family.

15. Identify factors that contribute to domestic violence.

16. How can the nurse care for a family that has experienced death?

17. What is a danger for a family with a rigid structure?

18. How can you assist individuals and families to avoid caregiver strain?

19. What effects does homelessness have on the health of the family?

Select the best answer for each of the following questions:

20. A nurse is working with a family in which the parents, both previously divorced, have brought a total of three unrelated children together. This type of family structure is classified as:
    1. nuclear.
    2. extended.
    3. blended.
    4. multiadult.

21. A community health nurse has been assigned to work with a patient who is being discharged from a psychiatric facility and returning to live with her parents. In planning care, the nurse recognizes that:
    1. family members do not need to understand and agree to the plan of care.
    2. health behaviors of the family do not influence the health of individual family members.
    3. a nurse needs to change the structure of the family to meet the needs of the patient.
    4. health promotion behaviors need to be tied to the developmental stage of the family.

22. Preparation for working with families includes understanding the life cycle stage that the patient is experiencing. A nurse is working with a family with young adults. It is expected that a family in this stage may also need to deal with:
    1. a review of life events.
    2. determining career goals.
    3. the death of an older parent.
    4. development of intimate peer relationships.

23. A nurse is working with a family that has been taking care of a parent with Alzheimer's disease for several years in their home. A nursing diagnosis of *potential for insufficient caregiver coping* is identified. The nurse initially plans for:
    1. respite care.
    2. more medication for the parent.
    3. placement in a long-term care facility.
    4. consultation with a family therapist.

24. After initial assessment of a family, a nurse determines that this is a healthy family. This assessment is based on the finding that:
    1. the family responds passively to stressors.
    2. change is viewed negatively and strongly resisted.
    3. the family structure is flexible enough to adapt to crises.
    4. minimum influence is exerted by the members upon their environment.

Copyright © 2019, Elsevier Inc. All Rights Reserved.

25. An older adult patient who had surgery is going to be discharged tomorrow. The patient has a visual deficit and will need dressing changes twice a day. To meet this specific need, the nurse first:
    1. refers the patient to an adult day care center.
    2. arranges for a private duty nurse to take care of the patient 24 hours a day.
    3. informs the patient that the dressing changes will have to be managed independently.
    4. investigates the availability of a family member or neighbor to perform the dressing changes.

26. A nurse is working in the community with an adult woman who is newly diagnosed with diabetes mellitus. The patient is married, has two school-age children, and works part time. The nurse is focused on assisting the patient to learn to manage the diabetes. At this point, the nurse is viewing the family as:
    1. patient.
    2. context.
    3. process.
    4. caregiver.

27. The concept of a family being able to actively deal with divorce and remarriage is termed:
    1. family context.
    2. family diversity.
    3. family hardiness.
    4. family functioning.

28. To determine family form and membership, a nurse asks the patient:
    1. "Who do you consider your family?"
    2. "Who drives the children to school?"
    3. "Where do you go on vacation?"
    4. "How are financial decisions made?"

29. The nurse is asking the family how the tasks are divided in the household. This question is used to establish the family's:
    1. structure.
    2. patterns.
    3. status.
    4. form.

30. Which is an accurate statement regarding characteristics of the "sandwich generation"?
    1. Usually the son or son-in-law is the family caregiver.
    2. The caregiver usually recognizes the need for and requests help.
    3. There is very little sense of responsibility for members of this group.
    4. The caregiver has conflicting responsibilities for aging parents, children, spouse, and job.

STUDY GROUP QUESTIONS

- What are the attributes of a family?
- What are the different family forms?
- What are the current challenges facing families?
- How do the structure and function of a family influence family relationships?
- How does communication affect family relationships?
- How are the nursing approaches to the family as patient and the family as context similar/different?
- How may critical thinking and nursing processes be applied to family nursing?
- What specific assessments should a nurse make in relation to a family?
- How does a nurse plan for the educational needs of a patient within a family?
- What must a nurse consider to meet the health needs of patients within families?
- How are psychosocial/cultural factors involved in family processes and the nursing approach to families?
- What resources are available within the health care setting and community to assist and support family functioning?

STUDY CHART

Create a study chart for your own family and identify the relationships among the members and each person's role and function.

Copyright © 2019, Elsevier Inc. All Rights Reserved.

26 Stress and Coping

PRELIMINARY READING

Chapter 26, pp. 663–681

CASE STUDIES

1. A young adult woman is preparing to be married in a few months. She has also received a recent job promotion that requires many additional hours to be spent at work. She is seen in a nurse practitioner's office for vague symptoms.
   a. What possible signs and symptoms may be demonstrated if this patient is experiencing a stress reaction?
   b. Identify a possible nursing diagnosis for this patient.
   c. Indicate an outcome for the nursing diagnosis.
   d. What relaxation techniques may be presented to this patient?

2. Mrs. C., 94 years old, lives alone in a one-story home in a senior housing community. Her neighbor and friend, who used to accompany her to the store and community events, died recently. Mrs. C. has had a recurrent upper respiratory infection, along with an arthritic right knee and worsening hearing loss. Her daughter lives an hour away and wants her to move into a senior development apartment nearby her.
   a. Identify the type of stressors that are having an impact upon Mrs. C.
   b. What are your priorities in working with Mrs. C.?

CHAPTER REVIEW

Complete the following:

1. Evaluating an event for its personal meaning is called:

2. Which of the following are correct statements about stress? Select all that apply.
   a. Increased self-confidence results in decreased tension. _____
   b. The emotional concern and support of others can increase negative effects. _____
   c. The same event can cause different stress levels in different people. _____
   d. The greater the perceived magnitude of the stressor, the greater the stress response. _____
   e. Stress is decreased if a person cannot anticipate the occurrence of an event. _____

3. A priority nursing intervention for safety for a patient under extreme stress is to determine:

4. Depression in later adulthood is a common problem.

   True _____ False _____

5. An example of a positive benefit of exercise for stress reduction is:

6. For the following, select the type of stress-producing factor that is indicated: *Situational, Maturational, Sociocultural*

   a. Divorce _____
   b. Poverty _____
   c. Immigration status _____
   d. Job change _____
   e. Adolescent identity crisis _____
   f. Hypertension _____
   g. Homelessness _____

7. Identify an indicator of stress for each of the following areas:
   a. Cognitive
   b. Cardiovascular
   c. Gastrointestinal
   d. Behavioral
   e. Neuroendocrine

Copyright © 2019, Elsevier Inc. All Rights Reserved.

8. a. Identify what stress management techniques can be taught to a patient.
   b. Indicate what strategies can be used to reduce stress for nurses.

9. Which of the following are signs of emotional stress? Select all that apply.

   a. Disruption of logical thinking _____

   b. Blaming others _____

   c. Good concentration _____

   d. Lack of interest _____

   e. Heightened creativity_____

   f. Attention to detail _____

   g. Irritability _____

10. Indicate an area that the nurse would discuss with the patient when using Pender's Health Promotion theory.

11. a. Compassion fatigue is most likely to be seen in a

    nurse who is working: _____
    (setting).
    b. What are the signs/symptoms of compassion fatigue?

12. In applying the QSEN competency of safety, what should the nurse assess in relation to stress and coping?

13. When does stress become a crisis?

14. The nurse is assessing a patient and is looking for outward indicators of stress. The following are objective signs associated with stress. Select all the apply.

   a. Twitching _____

   b. Hypotension _____

   c. Tachycardia _____

   d. Maintenance of eye contact _____

   e. Disheveled appearance _____

   f. Picking at the fingernails _____

15. Provide an example for each of the following:
   a. Developmental crisis

   b. Situational crisis

   c. Adventitious crisis

Select the best answer for each of the following questions:

16. A student who is coping by regressing will demonstrate which behavior?
   1. Becoming numb to the surroundings
   2. Refusing to discuss feelings
   3. Starting to act out in class
   4. Experiencing a loss of appetite

17. A patient has been hospitalized with a serious systemic infection. If the patient is in the resistance stage of the general adaptation syndrome and moving toward recovery, the nurse expects that the patient will demonstrate a:
   1. stabilization of hormone levels.
   2. greater degree of tissue damage.
   3. reduction in cardiac output.
   4. greater involvement of the sympathetic nervous system.

18. While working in a psychiatric emergency department, a nurse is alert to patients who are having severe difficulty in coping. A priority for the nurse is the safety of the patient and others; therefore, the nurse asks patients:
   1. "How can we help you?"
   2. "Are you thinking of harming yourself?"
   3. "What physical symptoms are you having?"
   4. "What happened that is different in your life?"

19. As a result of a patient's health problem, the family is experiencing economic difficulty and demonstrating signs of crisis. As part of crisis intervention, a nurse:
   1. refers the patient for financial assistance.
   2. recommends inpatient psychiatric therapy.
   3. plans to teach the family about long-term health needs.
   4. has the patient avoid discussions about personal feelings and emotions.

20. A nurse working for the surgical unit notes that a patient has been exhibiting nervous behavior the evening before a surgical procedure. To assess the degree of stress that the patient is experiencing, the nurse asks:
   1. "Would you like me to call your family for you?"
   2. "How dangerous do you think the surgery will be?"
   3. "You seem anxious. Would you like to talk about the surgery?"
   4. "How would you like to speak with another patient who has had the procedure already?"

Copyright © 2019, Elsevier Inc. All Rights Reserved.

21. A nurse identifies that a patient is experiencing a stress reaction. To determine how the patient may cope with the event, the nurse should ask:
    1. "Are you taking any hypnotics?"
    2. "What do you think caused your stress?"
    3. "How long have you felt this way?"
    4. "Have you dealt with this reaction before?"

22. An 80-year-old patient was admitted to the hospital with a diagnosis of pneumonia. The patient is very lethargic and not communicating, and the patient's respirations are extremely labored. The nurse assesses that the patient is experiencing the general adaptation stage of:
    1. alarm.
    2. resistance.
    3. exhaustion.
    4. reflex response.

23. A patient has gone to the employee support center with complaints of fatigue and general uneasiness. The patient believes that the symptoms may be related to the increased amount of work that is expected in the job. The nurse initially recommends that the patient should attempt to reduce or control the stress by:
    1. leaving the job immediately.
    2. enrolling in a self-awareness course.
    3. seeking the assistance of a psychiatrist.
    4. employing relaxation techniques, such as deep breathing.

24. According to general adaptation syndrome (GAS), a nurse expects which of the following signs as part of an alarm reaction?
    1. Pupil dilation
    2. Decreased blood glucose levels
    3. Decreased heart rate
    4. Stable hormone levels

25. A nurse identifies that a patient is under stress. To determine the patient's perception of the stress, the nurse should ask:
    1. "Are you sure you are not taking drugs or alcohol?"
    2. "What does the situation mean to you?"
    3. "How did you handle this in the past?"
    4. "Why aren't you seeing a counselor?"

26. Which of the following patient observations does a nurse associate with the ego-defense mechanism of conversion?
    1. Assuming more job responsibilities
    2. Having difficulty sleeping
    3. Acting out inappropriately
    4. Refusing to talk about a problem

27. A patient has been having a hard time at home. He goes outside and begins to yell about the car and starts kicking the tires. This is an example of which of the following ego-defense mechanisms?
    1. Displacement
    2. Compensation
    3. Identification
    4. Denial

28. A nurse wants to assess whether a patient is using maladaptive coping strategies. The patient should be asked specifically about his or her:
    1. dietary intake.
    2. social activities.
    3. cigarette smoking.
    4. exercise plan.

29. To determine a patient's available coping resources, a specific question to ask the patient is:
    1. "How often do you see your family members?"
    2. "How do you rate this life event?"
    3. "Has your appetite changed?"
    4. "Are you using alcohol or drugs?"

STUDY GROUP QUESTIONS

- What is stress?
- What theories are associated with stress and the stress response?
- How do nursing theorists explain stress and the stress response?
- How does the general adaptation syndrome (GAS) work?
- What factors influence the response to stress?
- What assessment data may indicate the presence of a stress reaction?
- How does stress relate to illness?
- What are coping/defense mechanisms, and how may they be used by individuals to deal with stress?
- What is the role of a nurse in reducing or eliminating stress for patients?
- What is involved in crisis intervention?
- What are possible relaxation/stress reduction techniques?

Copyright © 2019, Elsevier Inc. All Rights Reserved.

27 Loss and Grief

PRELIMINARY READING

Chapter 27, pp. 682–702

CASE STUDIES

1. A woman's husband committed suicide, and she is devastated by the event. In anticipation of potential difficulties, a nurse should be alert to the possibility of complicated grieving.
   a. What assessment data may indicate that the woman is experiencing a complicated period of bereavement?
   b. Identify a possible nursing diagnosis, goals, and nursing interventions for an individual who is experiencing complicated grieving.

2. The family tells the nurse that the patient is interested in hospice care. The siblings have questions about what services are available. As the nurse, what do you tell them about hospice care?

CHAPTER REVIEW

Match the description/definition in Column A with the correct term in Column B.

Column A	Column B
_____ 1. The emotional response to a loss	a. Actual loss
_____ 2. The conscious and unconscious behaviors associated with loss	b. Perceived loss
_____ 3. Recollection and re-experience of the deceased and the relationship by mentally or verbally reliving and remembering the person and past experiences	c. Situational loss
	d. Maturational loss
_____ 4. When a person can no longer touch, hear, see, or have valued people or objects	e. Reminiscence
_____ 5. The result of an unpredictable life event	f. Grief
_____ 6. A lifetime of normal developmental processes	g. Mourning
_____ 7. Loss that is uniquely experienced by a grieving person and often less obvious to others	

Complete the following:

8. Older adults are at risk for complicated grieving due to multiple losses, potential for cognitive impairment, or decreased physical abilities.

   True _____ False _____

9. Unexpected unemployment may be perceived as a loss.

   True _____ False _____

10. Provide an intervention that a nurse should implement for a family dealing with a patient's diagnosis of a terminal illness.

11. Which of the following interventions are appropriate for a terminally ill patient with constipation? Select all that apply.

    a. Maintenance of complete bed rest _____

    b. Increased intake of coffee _____

    c. Consumption of fresh vegetables _____

    d. Consumption of whole grain products _____

    e. Reducing fluid intake _____

    f. Obtaining an order for stool softeners _____

111

Copyright © 2019, Elsevier Inc. All Rights Reserved.

12. Identify at least two nursing measures that may be implemented to facilitate the mourning process.

13. Patients in the terminal stage of their lives may experience a sense of abandonment. What actions should a nurse implement to prevent or reduce this occurrence?

14. After a patient's death, there is federal and state legislation regarding policies and procedures for:

15. Formulate a question that a nurse could ask a patient regarding:
    a. The nature of a loss:
    b. His/her cultural beliefs about loss:
    c. How the family is coping with the loss:

16. A patient has been in hospice care at home. A family member is taking care of the patient and is concerned about the patient's impending death, particularly what will happen to the patient. The nurse informs the family member that the signs of impending death include:

17. a. According to Worden, moving through the four tasks typically takes _____ (time frame).

    b. Identify Worden's four tasks:

18. What are the 'R's in Rando's R Process Model?

19. In performing postmorten care, which are the correct actions? Select all that apply.
    a. Position the patient upright at 45-90 degrees. _____
    b. Ask the family members if they want to help with the care. _____
    c. Discard remaining personal items. _____
    d. Close the patient's eyes. _____
    e. Leave dentures in the patient's mouth. _____
    f. Remove all of the tubes and devices before an autopsy is performed. _____

20. Identify nursing interventions for the following symptoms that may be experienced by a patient who is dying.
    a. Fatigue:

    b. Decreased appetite:

    c. Nausea:

21. Identify five examples of physical sensations or behaviors that may be observed with normal grieving.

22. When would an autopsy be expected to be performed?

23. Identify what should be included in the documentation following a patient's death.

24. Identify general factors that may influence loss or grief.

25. For the QSEN Competency of Teamwork and Collaboration, what other referrals or consultations may be indicated for a patient who is terminally ill?

26. How do modern theories of grief differ from earlier theories?

27. What specific communication may promote hope and help the patient to explore goals, worth, and adaptations to future changes?

Select the best answer for each of the following questions:

28. A nurse is working with a patient who has been diagnosed with a terminal disease. The patient, who is moving into Kübler-Ross's denial stage of grieving, may respond:
    1. "I understand what the diagnosis means, and I know that I may die."
    2. "I would like to be able to make it to my son's wedding in June."
    3. "I think that the diagnostic tests are wrong, and they should be redone."
    4. "I don't think that I can stand to have any more treatments. I just want to feel better."

Copyright © 2019, Elsevier Inc. All Rights Reserved.

29. While working with young children in a day care center, a nurse responds to instances that occur in their lives. Toddlers at the center generally experience loss and grief associated with:
    1. anticipation of loss.
    2. separation from parents.
    3. changes in physical abilities.
    4. development of their identities.

30. In a senior citizen center, a nurse is talking with a group of older adults. The recurrent theme associated with loss for this age group is a:
    1. confusion of fact and fantasy.
    2. perceived threat to their identity.
    3. change in status, role, and lifestyle.
    4. determination to reexamine life goals.

31. A nurse who has recently graduated from nursing school is employed by an oncology unit. There are a number of patients who will not improve and will need assistance with dying. The nurse prepares for this experience by:
    1. completing a detailed course on legal aspects of end of life issues.
    2. controlling his or her emotions about dying patients.
    3. experiencing the death of a close family member.
    4. identifying his or her own feelings about death and dying.

32. A patient has had a long illness and is now approaching the end stages of his life. To assist this patient to meet his need for self-worth and support during this time, the nurse:
    1. arranges for a grief counselor to visit.
    2. leaves the patient alone to deal with his life issues.
    3. asks the patient's family to take over his care.
    4. plans to visit the patient regularly throughout the day.

33. The spouse of a patient who has just died is having more frequent episodes of headaches and generalized joint pain. The initial nursing intervention for this individual is to:
    1. complete a thorough pain assessment.
    2. encourage more frequent use of analgesics.
    3. sit with the patient and encourage discussion of feelings.
    4. refer the patient immediately to a psychologist or grief counselor.

34. A patient is experiencing a very serious illness that may not be curable. The nurse promotes hope for this patient when:
    1. establishing firm goals.
    2. encouraging the development of supportive relationships.
    3. withholding information about the illness and its treatment.
    4. referring the patient for psychological counseling.

35. A patient in the long-term care facility is to receive palliative care measures only during the end stages of a terminal illness. The nurse anticipates that this will include:
    1. pain relief measures.
    2. emergency surgery.
    3. pulmonary resuscitation.
    4. transfer to intensive care if necessary.

36. A patient arrives for outpatient chemotherapy. During this visit the patient tells the nurse that she is experiencing periods of nausea. The nurse promotes patient comfort by providing:
    1. milk.
    2. coffee.
    3. ginger ale.
    4. orange juice.

37. The loss of a known environment is associated with:
    1. being hospitalized for several days.
    2. the death of a pet.
    3. amputation of the right leg.
    4. a recent burglary in the home.

38. Of the following, a situational loss occurs when a:
    1. parent requires physical assistance.
    2. family friend dies.
    3. child goes to college.
    4. job demotion and pay reduction occur.

39. An individual in Bowlby's second phase of mourning, yearning, and searching may be expected to:
    1. be unable to believe the loss.
    2. endlessly examine how the loss occurred.
    3. acquire new skills and build new relationships.
    4. experience emotional outbursts and sobbing.

40. A nurse recognizes anticipatory grief in the person who:
    1. has an active period of mourning that does not decrease and continues over time.
    2. cannot function and is overwhelmed, with resulting substance abuse or phobias.
    3. accepts the reality of a terminal diagnosis and begins to say goodbye and complete life affairs before death occurs.
    4. is not aware that behaviors are interfering with daily activities, such as sleeping and eating.

41. The nurse is using Worden's Four Tasks of Mourning to assess the family member's response to the death of a loved one. What is expected when the individual moves into Task III, *Adjust to the environment in which the deceased is missing*?
    1. Realizing that the loved one is gone.
    2. Taking on roles of the loved one.
    3. Suppressing feelings over the loss.
    4. Forgetting the deceased and moving on.

Copyright © 2019, Elsevier Inc. All Rights Reserved.

STUDY GROUP QUESTIONS

- What are loss and grief?
- What are the different types of grief and possible reactions to these losses?
- What are the differences and similarities between the theories of grief and loss?
- How may the grieving process be influenced by special circumstances?
- How are hope, spirituality, and self-concept related to loss and grieving?
- What behaviors are associated with loss and grieving?
- What resources are available for patient, family, and nurse that assist in the grieving process?
- What principles facilitate mourning?
- How may a nurse apply critical thinking and nursing processes to the patient/family experiencing loss and grieving?
- How are religious and cultural beliefs associated with loss, grief, death, and dying?
- How may a nurse intervene to assist a patient/family with loss and the grieving process?
- What is involved in care of the body after death?

Copyright © 2019, Elsevier Inc. All Rights Reserved.

28 Activity and Exercise

PRELIMINARY READING

Chapter 28, pp. 703–740

CASE STUDY

1. A nurse is assigned to work with an 80-year-old woman residing in a nursing home. There is conflicting information in the chart about her ability to move around independently. The nurse is concerned about meeting the patient's needs for proper body mechanics as well as her safety.
   a. What important assessment information is needed to plan meeting the patient's needs?
   b. If the patient is unable to ambulate independently, what nursing interventions should be planned?

CHAPTER REVIEW

Match the description/definition in Column A with the correct term in Column B.

	Column A	*Column B*
_____	1. Awareness of the position of the body and its parts	a. Body mechanics
_____	2. Resistance that a moving body meets from the surface on which it moves	b. Ergonomics
_____	3. Manner or style of walking	c. Range of motion
_____	4. Lying face up	d. Posture
_____	5. The design of work tasks to best suit the capabilities of workers	e. Alignment
_____	6. The relationship of one body part to another along a horizontal or vertical line	f. Supine
_____	7. Maintenance of optimal body position	g. Friction
_____	8. Body alignment during walking, turning, lifting, or carrying	h. Gait
_____	9. Mobility of the joint	i. Proprioception

Complete the following:

10. Identify at least three components to assess to determine a patient's mobility.

11. Which of the following are correct principles of body mechanics? Select all that apply.

    a. Maintain a narrow base of support. _____

    b. Face the direction of movement. _____

    c. Maintain a higher center of gravity. _____

    d. Divide balanced activity between the arms and legs. _____

    e. Increase friction between the object and surface. _____

    f. Alternate periods of rest and activity. _____

12. The best way to determine a patient's level of pain is to observe for redness or swelling of the joints.

    True _____ False _____

115

Copyright © 2019, Elsevier Inc. All Rights Reserved.

13. For a patient who has been on prolonged bed rest:
    a. What should the nurse do to prepare the patient before ambulation?

    b. Transfers and position changes for this patient can lead to the development of: _____

    _____

14. Identify at least two pathological influences on alignment, exercise, or activity.

15. Range of motion can be determined by observing the patient's gait and ability to perform activities of daily living.

    True _____ False _____

16. An example of a physiological factor that may influence activity tolerance is:

17. Identify a nursing diagnosis associated with a change in a patient's ability to maintain physical activity.

18. For a patient who has severe arthritis and is unable to perform activities of daily living because of discomfort on movement, the priority is to:

19. What aspects of the patient's gait are assessed by the nurse?

20. Complete the following about transferring patients.
    a. The general "rule of thumb" for transfers is:

    b. A nurse's priority during patient transfers is:

21. How does the nurse determine a patient's activity tolerance?

22. Which of the following are expected findings for assessment of a patient while standing? Select all that apply.

    a. Head is erect and held midline. _____

    b. Body parts are asymmetrical. _____

    c. The spine has a lateral curve. _____

    d. The abdomen protrudes. _____

    e. The knees are in a straight line between the hips and ankles. _____

    f. The feet are pointed at an angle and close together. _____

    g. The arms hang comfortably at the sides. _____

23. Which of the following indicate correct care or technique for a patient who is using crutches? Select all that apply.

    a. The patient leans on the axillae to support his or her weight. _____

    b. Both crutches are transferred to one hand when preparing to sit. _____

    c. Crutches are placed 1 (one) foot to the front and side of the feet. _____

    d. The patient has a non–weight-bearing left leg and is using a three-point gait. _____

    e. The unaffected leg is advanced first when the patient goes up the stairs. _____

24. Patients who are on prolonged bed rest need to be repositioned at least every _____ hours.

25. a. When transferring patients who are able to assist from the bed to a chair, the chair should be positioned:

    b. Identify the steps, in order, for the use of a mechanical lift.

26. Logrolling a patient in bed requires at least _____ caregivers to perform.

27. A nurse observes a patient and notes that there is limited range of motion in a few areas. This could be the result of:

28. The patient, who has some mobility in the upper arms and legs, needs to be moved up in bed. What should the nurse do to reduce friction when moving the patient?

29. Half of all back pain is associated with:

30. Improper positioning of patients in bed can lead to:

31. A mechanical device that is used for specific repetitive joint exercise is a:

Copyright © 2019, Elsevier Inc. All Rights Reserved.

32. Identify at least three components of a safe patient-handling program.

33. a. More than 45% of adults aged 45-54 meet the national activity guidelines.

    True _____ False _____

    b. Sociocultural factors have an impact upon the amount of physical activity that is done by an individual.

    True _____ False _____

34. Which of the following are positive effects of exercise? Select all that apply.

    a. Increased fatigue _____

    b. Improved muscle tone _____

    c. Reduced bone loss _____

    d. Decreased cardiac output _____

    e. Increased production of body heat _____

    f. Decreased use of glucose and fatty acids _____

Select the best answer for each of the following questions:

35. A patient is able to bear weight on one foot. The crutch-walking gait that the nurse teaches this patient is the:
    1. two-point gait.
    2. swing-through gait.
    3. three-point alternating gait.
    4. four-point alternating gait.

36. A nurse is working with a patient who is able only to assist the nurse in moving from the bed to the chair. The nurse needs to help the patient to stand. The correct technique for lifting the patient to stand and pivot to the chair is for the nurse to:
    1. keep the legs straight.
    2. maintain a wide base with the feet.
    3. keep the stomach muscles loose.
    4. support the patient away from the body.

37. A patient has experienced an injury to his lower extremity. The orthopedist has prescribed the use of crutches and a four-point gait. The nurse instructs the patient using this gait to:
    1. move the right crutch forward first.
    2. move both crutches forward together.
    3. move the right foot and the left crutch together.
    4. move the right foot and the right crutch together.

38. The patient had a cerebrovascular accident (CVA/stroke) with resultant left hemiparesis. The nurse is instructing the patient on the use of a cane for support during ambulation. The nurse instructs the patient to:
    1. use the cane on the right side.
    2. use the cane on the left side.
    3. move the left foot forward first.
    4. move the right foot forward first.

39. A patient is admitted to the rehabilitation facility for physical therapy after an automobile accident. To conduct an assessment of the patient's body alignment, the nurse should begin by:
    1. observing the patient's gait.
    2. explaining the process.
    3. determining the level of activity tolerance.
    4. evaluating the full extent of joint range of motion.

40. An average-size female patient who resides in the extended care facility requires assistance to ambulate down the hall. The nurse has noticed that the patient has some weakness on her right side. The nurse assists this patient to ambulate by:
    1. standing at the patient's left side and holding her arm.
    2. walking in front of her and having her hold onto her waist.
    3. standing behind her and encircling one arm around the patient's waist.
    4. standing at her right side and using a gait belt.

41. A patient has a cast on the right foot and is being discharged home. Crutches will be used for ambulation, and the patient has stairs to manage to enter the house and to get to the bedroom and bathroom. The nurse observes that the patient is not that confident with the use of the crutches, so plans to teach the patient to use which of the following techniques for the stairs?
    1. Advance the crutches first to ascend the stairs.
    2. Use one crutch for support while going up and down.
    3. Sit on the stairs and lift with the arms and weight-bearing leg to move up.
    4. Use the banister or wall for support when descending the stairs.

42. A patient is getting up to ambulate for the first time since a surgical procedure. While ambulating in the hallway, the patient complains of severe dizziness. The nurse should first:
    1. call for help.
    2. lower the patient gently to the floor.
    3. lean the patient against the wall until the episode passes.
    4. support the patient and move quickly back to the room.

117

Copyright © 2019, Elsevier Inc. All Rights Reserved.

43. One of the expected benefits of exercise is:
    1. decreased diaphragmatic excursion.
    2. decreased cardiac output.
    3. decreased resting heart rate.
    4. increased fatigue.

44. A nurse selects which of the following for promoting resistive isometric exercise for a patient?
    1. Whirlpool
    2. Footboard
    3. Weights
    4. Stationary bicycle

45. The first step in initiating an exercise program for a patient is to:
    1. select the equipment.
    2. design the fitness program.
    3. schedule time during the day.
    4. seek approval from the health care prescriber.

46. An expected assessment of a toddler's alignment will indicate a:
    1. slight swayback and protruding abdomen.
    2. flexed spine without anteroposterior curves.
    3. full musculoskeletal function and straight posture.
    4. distinct thoracic curvature and weakness.

47. For inpatient early progressive mobility, Level 3 includes beginning to have the patient:
    1. sitting in bed with the head of the bed or stretcher elevated to 45 degrees.
    2. sitting on the edge of the bed.
    3. actively transferring to a chair.
    4. initiating ambulation.

48. Which of the following assessment findings indicates that exercise should be discontinued?
    a. Heart rate = 145 beats/minute
    b. Blood pressure 140/82
    c. Respirations 32 breaths/minute
    d. Oxygen saturation 95%

49. What is the proper alignment for a patient in the sitting position?
    1. Body weight distributed totally to the buttocks.
    2. Both feet supported on the floor.
    3. Head flexed forward at a 60-degree angle.
    4. A 10" space maintained between the edge of the seat and the popliteal space.

STUDY GROUP QUESTIONS

- What are body mechanics?
- How is body movement regulated by the musculoskeletal and nervous systems?
- What general changes occur in the body's appearance and function throughout growth and development?
- How can body mechanics be influenced by pathological conditions?
- What patient assessment data should be obtained regarding body mechanics?
- What is activity tolerance?
- How can proper body mechanics be promoted for patients in different health care settings?
- What safety measures should be implemented before patient transfers and ambulation?
- What are the proper procedures for exercises, transfers, and ambulation?
- How should a patient be instructed to use assistive devices, such as canes, walkers, and crutches?

STUDY CHART

Create a study chart to describe how to *Safely Use Assistive Devices for Ambulation* that identifies the nursing actions and patient instruction required to reduce possible hazards for the following devices: gait belt, cane, walker, crutches.

Copyright © 2019, Elsevier Inc. All Rights Reserved.

29 Immobility

Chapter 29, pp. 741–781

CASE STUDIES

1. A patient has just gone to the rehabilitation facility. She has been immobilized with a spinal cord injury from an automobile accident. You are aware of the physical hazards of immobility, but her withdrawn behavior is your concern now.
   a. What can you do to prevent the possible psychological and emotional effects of the patient's period of immobility?

2. A patient will be getting out of bed for the first time after having surgery and receiving general anesthesia.
   a. What actions should be taken by the nurse to promote the patient's safety?

3. You are the nurse in a long-term care facility and your assignment includes several older adult patients who are immobile.
   a. What actions should be taken specifically for this older adult population?

CHAPTER REVIEW

Match the descriptions/definitions in Column A with the correct term in Column B.

Column A

_____ 1. Characterized by bone resorption

_____ 2. Temporary decrease in blood supply to an organ or tissue.

_____ 3. Capacity to maneuver around freely

_____ 4. Permanent plantar flexion

_____ 5. Lung inflammation from stasis or pooling of secretions

_____ 6. Increased urine excretion

_____ 7. Collapse of alveoli

_____ 8. Bathing, dressing, eating

_____ 9. Calcium stones in the kidney

_____ 10. Accumulation of platelets, fibrin, clotting factors, and cellular elements attached to the interior wall of an artery or vein

Column B

a. Renal calculi

b. Diuresis

c. Hypostatic pneumonia

d. Mobility

e. Ischemia

f. Atelectasis

g. Thrombus

h. Activities of daily living

i. Disuse osteoporosis

j. Footdrop

Complete the following:

11. The objectives or advantages of bed rest are:

12. Identify the four pathological influences on mobility and an example of each one.

119

13. Which of the following pathophysiological changes occur with immobility? Select all that apply.

  a. Increased basal metabolic rate _____

  b. Decreased gastrointestinal motility _____

  c. Orthostatic hypotension _____

  d. Increased appetite _____

  e. Increased oxygen availability _____

  f. Hypercalcemia _____

  g. Increased lung expansion _____

  h. Decreased cardiac output _____

  i. Increased dependent edema _____

  j. Decreased stressors _____

  k. Increased urinary stasis _____

  l. Decreased passive behaviors _____

14. An example of a fluid and electrolyte imbalance that may occur with prolonged immobility is:

15. An example of a common behavioral change that may be observed in an immobilized patient is:

16. A nurse anticipates that a patient on prolonged bed rest will have an increased heart rate.

  True _____   False _____

17. The Virchow triad is related to _____

  _____, and the three associated

  problems are: _____

18. With an immobilized child, the nurse's focus is on:

19. An important concept when working with patients who are immobilized is to maintain the patient's autonomy. The nurse can accomplish this by:

20. Identify the following positions for patients:

  a. _____

  b. _____

  c. _____

21. Identify at least one major change that may occur in each of the following body systems as a result of immobility and a nursing intervention to prevent or treat the change.

  a. Cardiovascular

  b. Respiratory

  c. Integumentary

  d. Gastrointestinal

  e. Urinary

  f. Musculoskeletal

22. Using the algorithm for patient transfers, the appropriate intervention for a patient who is cooperative, has upper body strength, but cannot bear full weight should be:

23. What areas are included in a focused patient assessment of overall mobility?

Copyright © 2019, Elsevier Inc. All Rights Reserved.

24. Identify for each of the following illustrations what range-of-joint-motion (ROJM) exercise is being performed:
a.

b.

c.

d.

e.

25. To reduce extension of the fingers and abduction

of the thumb, the nurse should use _____

_____ when positioning the patient.

26. Where should a nurse check for edema in an immobilized patient?

27. For an immobilized patient, identify the usual frequency of assessment for the following:
a. Respiratory status:
b. Anorexia:
c. Urinary elimination:
d. Total intake and output:

28. What are anthropometric measurements and how often are they assessed?

29. Specific range of motion exercises to prevent thrombophlebitis include:

30. For a patient who will have antiembolic stockings:
a. The contraindications for their use are:
b. How often are they are removed?
c. A nurse makes sure that the stockings are NOT:
d. Application of the stockings may be delegated to an unlicensed nursing assistant.

   True _____ False _____

31. Which of the following actions are correct for the use of a sequential compression device? Select all that apply.
a. The back of the patient's ankle and knee are

   aligned with markings on the sleeve. _____

b. A hand width is left between the sleeve and the

   patient's skin. _____

c. The sleeve and device are removed once daily.

   _____

d. The unit is observed through one complete cycle

   after application. _____

e. A small amount of powder or cornstarch can be

   applied to the legs if not sensitive. _____

f. Allow patient to ambulate with SCD or MCD.

   _____

32. a. A medication that is used to reduce the risk of thrombophlebitis is:

b. It is usually given every _____ hours by the

   _____ route.

33. Pain can interfere with a patient's activity. How would you assess a patient's pain and observe for signs of pain?

34. For a patient who had a cerebrovascular accident (CVA, or stroke) with right-sided hemiplegia, identify how the patient can be involved in performing joint range of motion exercise.

35. Identify measures to prevent pressure injuries.

121

Copyright © 2019, Elsevier Inc. All Rights Reserved.

36. Identify a nursing diagnosis for a patient who is immobilized.

37. a. The patient has a reddened area on the coccyx/buttocks. The nurse considers positioning the patient in:

    b. For the patient with acute respiratory distress, the best position is:

    c. The patient is too weak to cough. What will be necessary to maintain the airway?

    d. For the chair-bound patient, the patient should move:

38. Put the following steps in order for preparing to move the patient in bed.

    a. Raise the level of the bed to a comfortable working height. _____

    b. Close the door to the room. _____

    c. Determine the number of people needed to assist. _____

    d. Perform hand hygiene. _____

    e. Explain the procedure to the patient. _____

    f. Obtain equipment. _____

39. What is included in thromboprophylaxis?

Select the best answer for each of the following questions:

40. After a CVA (stroke) a patient is prescribed prolonged bed rest. During assessment, the nurse is especially alert to the presence of:
    1. an increased joint ROM.
    2. an increased hemoglobin level.
    3. an increased muscle mass.
    4. a unilateral increase in calf circumference.

41. For a patient who has been placed in a spica (full body) cast, the nurse remains alert to possible changes in the cardiovascular system as a result of immobility. The nurse may find that the patient has:
    1. hypertension.
    2. tachycardia.
    3. hypervolemia.
    4. an increased cardiac output.

42. A possible complication for a patient who has been prescribed prolonged bed rest is thrombus formation. For the nurse to assess the presence of this serious problem, the nurse should:
    1. attempt to elicit Chvostek sign.
    2. palpate the temperature of the feet.
    3. measure the patient's calf and thigh diameters.
    4. observe for hair loss and skin turgor in the lower legs.

43. A patient was prescribed extended bed rest after abdominal surgery. The patient now has an order to be out of bed. The nurse should first:
    1. assess respiratory function.
    2. take the patient's blood pressure.
    3. ask if the patient feels light-headed.
    4. assist the patient to the edge of the bed.

44. A patient has been placed in skeletal traction and will be immobilized for an extended period of time. The nurse recognizes that there is a need to prevent respiratory complications and intervenes by:
    1. suctioning the airway every hour.
    2. changing the patient's position every 4–8 hours.
    3. using oxygen and nebulizer treatments regularly.
    4. encouraging deep breathing and coughing every hour.

45. Patients who are immobilized in health care facilities require that their psychosocial needs be met along with their physiological needs. A nurse recognizes a patient's psychosocial needs when telling the patient the following:
    1. "The staff will limit your visitors so that you will not be bothered."
    2. "We will help you get dressed so you can look more presentable."
    3. "We can discuss the routine to see if there are any changes that you may want to make."
    4. "A roommate can sometimes be a real bother and very distracting. We can move you to a private room."

46. A patient is transferred to a rehabilitation facility from the medical center after a CVA (stroke). The CVA resulted in severe right-sided paralysis, and the patient is very limited in mobility. To prevent the complication of external hip rotation for this patient, the nurse uses a:
    1. footboard.
    2. bed board.
    3. trapeze bar.
    4. trochanter roll.

Copyright © 2019, Elsevier Inc. All Rights Reserved.

47. A patient who has deep vein thrombosis is at risk for:
    1. atelectasis.
    2. pulmonary emboli.
    3. orthostatic hypotension.
    4. hypostatic pneumonia.

48. The equipment that is used on a bed to assist a patient to raise the torso is a:
    1. sandbag.
    2. bed board.
    3. trapeze bar.
    4. wedge pillow.

49. For exercise, which of the following is appropriate for an immobilized older adult?
    1. Gradual, extended warm-ups
    2. Rapid transitions and movements
    3. Sustained isometric exercises
    4. Increased intensity programs

50. If all of the following are prescribed, the best nursing strategy for the prevention of renal calculi is:
    1. administration of diuretics.
    2. provision of a high-fiber diet.
    3. insertion of a urinary catheter.
    4. offering of 2 liters of fluid per day.

51. A nurse is instructing a patient on joint range of motion and performance of shoulder extension. The nurse correctly instructs the patient to:
    1. raise the arm straight forward.
    2. straighten the elbow by lowering the hand.
    3. rotate the arm until the thumb is turned inward and toward the back.
    4. move the arm behind the body with the elbow straight.

52. To prevent plantar flexion, a nurse will obtain:
    1. trochanter rolls.
    2. foot boots.
    3. sandbags.
    4. hand splints.

53. A nurse is instructing a patient on range of motion and performance of forearm supination. The nurse correctly instructs the patient to:
    1. move the palm toward the inner aspect of the forearm.
    2. turn the lower arm and hand so the palm is up.
    3. straighten the elbow by lowering the hand.
    4. touch the thumb to each finger of the hand.

54. A patient has weakness to the upper and lower extremities and has been on bed rest for several days. Which of the following actions performed by the new staff nurse requires correction?
    1. Performing passive range of motion exercises
    2. Having the patient do as much of the bath as possible
    3. Massaging the lower extremities
    4. Assisting the patient to different positions every 1½ hours

55. A patient is being instructed to perform dorsal flexion of the foot. The nurse observes the patient's ability to:
    1. turn the foot and leg toward the other leg.
    2. move the foot so the toes point upward.
    3. turn the sole of the foot medially.
    4. straighten and spread the toes of the foot.

56. The nurse is applying a sequential compression device on the immobilized patient. Which of the following actions is appropriate?
    1. Make sure the red light is on so the unit will run.
    2. Remove the device after 2–3 days.
    3. Check for function after 10 or more complete cycles.
    4. Fit two fingers between the patient's leg and the device sleeve.

57. A nurse selects which of the following for maintaining dorsal flexion for the patient?
    1. Pillows
    2. Foot boots
    3. Bed boards
    4. Trochanter rolls

58. A nurse recognizes that the position that is **contraindicated** for a patient who is at risk for aspiration is:
    1. Fowler's.
    2. lateral.
    3. Sims.
    4. supine.

59. A patient had total hip replacement surgery and requires careful postoperative positioning to maintain the legs in abduction. The nurse will obtain a:
    1. foot boot.
    2. trapeze bar.
    3. bed board.
    4. wedge pillow.

Copyright © 2019, Elsevier Inc. All Rights Reserved.

60. The nurse documents that the patient has lordosis because which of the following was observed?
    1. An exaggeration of the anterior convex curve of the lumbar spine
    2. An increased convexity in the curvature of the thoracic spine
    3. Inclining of the head to the affected side where the sternocleidomastoid muscle is contracted
    4. Lateral S- or C-shaped spinal column with vertebral rotation and unequal heights of the hips and shoulders

STUDY GROUP QUESTIONS

- What are the basic concepts of mobility?
- What is immobility?
- How is bed rest used therapeutically?
- What physiological changes may occur throughout the body as a result of immobility?
- What psychosocial and developmental changes may occur as a result of immobility?
- What assessments should be made by a nurse to determine the effect of immobility on the patient?
- What nursing interventions should be implemented to prevent or treat the effects of immobility?

Copyright © 2019, Elsevier Inc. All Rights Reserved.

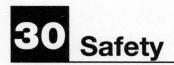 **Safety**

PRELIMINARY READING

Chapter 30, pp. 782–811

CASE STUDIES

1. You will be accompanying the visiting nurse to the home of a family with two young children who are ages 2 and 4 years.
   a. What general assessment information should be obtained regarding home safety during the visit?
   b. What specific safety observations should be made because there are two young children residing in the home?

2. A patient with diabetes mellitus is living at home and needs to take daily insulin injections.
   a. What are some of the precautions that this patient should take to avoid pathogen transmission and maintain safety?

3. You are currently working in a long-term care facility. There are a number of patients who are recognized as being at risk for falls. A restraint-free environment is desired.
   a. What specific interventions may be implemented to prevent falls and provide for patient safety without the use of restraints?

4. Upon home assessment, the nurse finds that the patient and her husband have accumulated years of newspapers that they have placed into multiple piles throughout the main living area. This has created a maze-like environment that makes it very difficult when they are trying to move around.
   a. Identify nursing diagnoses, goals, and nursing interventions that are applicable to this patient's situation.

CHAPTER REVIEW

Complete the following:

1. What are some examples that might affect these basic needs?
   a. Oxygen:
   b. Nutrition:
   c. Temperature:

2. Provide an example of a possible physical hazard that may be found in the home.

3. For older adults:
   a. Identify at least three physiological changes that increase the risk of accidents for older adults:
   b. Indicate at least two areas that should be included in teaching the older adult about:
      (1) Driving safety
      (2) Home environment safety

4. For each of the following, identify a nursing intervention that may be implemented to prevent injury and promote patient safety.
   a. Falls:
   b. Patient-inherent accidents:
   c. Procedure-related risks:
   d. Equipment-related risks:

5. The Centers for Medicare and Medicaid Services (CMS) have identified that payment will be denied for events that are not present on admission but occur during hospitalization. Which of the following are included in the CMS listing of these occurrences? Select all that apply.

   a. Air embolism _____

   b. Blood transfusion _____

   c. Patient falls _____

   d. Wrong medication administered _____

   e. Surgical site infection _____

   f. Stage III pressure ulcer _____

Copyright © 2019, Elsevier Inc. All Rights Reserved.

6. Immunity that occurs as a result of injection of a small amount of weakened or dead organisms and modified toxins is called:

7. For each of the following age groups, identify an example of a potential safety hazard and instruction that can be provided.
   a. Infant, toddler, preschooler:
   b. School age child:
   c. Adolescent:
   d. Adult:
   e. Older adult:

8. During an assessment, a nurse determines that a patient with a high risk for injury is an individual experiencing:

9. Identify which of the following are intrinsic factors that contribute to a patient's risk for falling. Select all that apply.

   a. Age 65 or older. _____

   b. Loose electrical cords. _____

   c. Liquid spilled on the floor. _____

   d. Limited visual acuity. _____

   e. Clutter between the bed and bathroom. _____

   f. Poor balance. _____

   g. Orthostatic hypotension. _____

10. There is a greater risk for poisoning as a result of finding multiple medications in the home of an older adult.

    True _____ False _____

11. a. A restraint is defined as:

    b. Chemical restraints are:

12. The primary goal when using restraints (safety reminder devices) is to:

13. A restraint is indicated for a patient in the hospital. Which of the following are correct for the use of restraints? Select all that apply.
    a. Obtain renewals for restraint orders every 72 hours.

    _____

    b. Evaluate the patient at least every 1–2 hours.

    _____

c. Pad the skin under the restraint. _____

d. Keep the restraint in place for 8 hours. _____

e. At least two fingers should fit under the secured restraint. _____

f. Tie the restraint ends with a knot. _____

g. Attach the restraint ties to the side rails. _____

14. Side rails may be used at any time to keep a patient in bed.

    True _____ False _____

15. An older adult patient who often forgets to take medication or does not remember if it was taken may benefit from a(n):

16. Identify an example of a medication safety strategy that is used in a health care agency.

17. For the following areas, identify a specific environmental adjustment that should be made to promote safety.
    a. Tactile deficit:
    b. Visual deficit:

18. Among adults 65 years and older, falls in the home are the leading cause of unintentional death.

    True _____ False _____

19. a. You know that a piece of equipment in the acute care agency is safe to use when:
    b. Health care providers are exposed to possible poisons in the acute care environment by:

20. Carbon monoxide poisoning can occur in the home.
    a. Identify the signs and symptoms associated with low concentrations.
    b. What safety measure is necessary to prevent exposure?

21. Explain the "Speak Up" campaign.

22. What resources/agencies are available for patient safety standards?

23. What are the leading causes of falls in the home?

Copyright © 2019, Elsevier Inc. All Rights Reserved.

24. Information about chemical substances in the health care workplace can be found in:

25. The parents of an adolescent are concerned about possible substance abuse. What signs, symptoms, and behaviors are indicative of this problem?

26. For disaster management, hospitals are required to have what resources in place?

27. The application of physical restraints may be delegated to nursing assistive personnel.

    True _____ False _____

28. Identify the meaning of the following for fire management:

    R: P:
    A: A:
    C: S:
    E: S:

29. Match the type of fire extinguisher with the form of fire. Type A, Type B, Type C

    a. Grease fire _____

    b. Electrical fire _____

    c. Paper fire _____

30. The nurse notices that the plug for the infusion pump makes a spark when it is plugged into the wall socket. The nurse should:

31. Identify at least one (1) Patient Safety Goal identified by The Joint Commission for the following:
    a. Hospitals
    b. Home care

32. Place the steps for the Timed Get Up and Go Test in order:

    a. Stand still momentarily _____

    b. Sit down _____

    c. Walk 10 feet (3 meters) (in a line) _____

    d. Turn around _____

    e. Stand up from the arm chair _____

    f. Walk back to chair _____

    g. Turn around _____

    What is an abnormal result for the test?

33. Indicate safety measures for the following:
    a. Use of home oxygen
    b. Food preparation

34. For the following patient scenario, identify the assessment findings that the nurse should focus on to prevent patient injuries.

    Upon entering the patient's home, the visiting nurse observed that the patient was wearing slippers with no back slip-ons. The patient stated that she seemed to always leave her glasses somewhere. There were piles of newspapers and other items cluttering the floor around the living room chairs. The lighting in the stairway was less than 60, watts and there were throw rugs on the wood floors in the halls. When looking through the medicine cabinet with the patient, the nurse noted that some medications were expired. The patient admitted to falling once when getting up during the night to go to the bathroom.

Select the best answer for each of the following questions:

35. The nurse recognizes the importance of teaching the patient who is using oxygen at home that the leading cause of burns and fires is:
    1. smoking.
    2. the use of heating blankets.
    3. the misuse of the stove.
    4. damage to the oxygen tank.

36. An older adult patient is being discharged home. The patient will be taking furosemide (Lasix) on a daily basis. A specific consideration for this patient is:
    1. exposure to the sun.
    2. the location of the bathroom.
    3. food consumption when taking the medication.
    4. financial considerations for long-term care.

37. While walking through a hallway in the extended care facility, a nurse notices smoke coming from a wastebasket in a patient's room. Upon closer investigation, the nurse identifies that there is a fire that is starting to flare up. The nurse should first:
    1. extinguish the fire.
    2. remove the patient from the room.
    3. contain the fire by closing the door to the room.
    4. turn off all of the surrounding electrical equipment.

38. A patient is newly admitted to the hospital and appears to be disoriented. There is a concern for the patient's immediate safety. The nurse is considering the use of restraints to prevent an injury. The nurse recognizes that the use of restraints in a hospital requires:
    1. a physician's order.
    2. the patient's consent.
    3. a family member's consent.
    4. agreement among the nursing staff.

127

Copyright © 2019, Elsevier Inc. All Rights Reserved.

39. A nurse is completing admission histories for newly admitted patients to the unit. The nurse is aware that the patient with the greatest risk of injury:
    1. is 84 years of age.
    2. uses corrective lenses.
    3. has a history of falls.
    4. has arthritis in the lower extremities.

40. A child has ingested a poisonous substance. The parent is instructed by the nurse to:
    1. take the child to the hospital immediately.
    2. administer 30 mL of emetic.
    3. take the child to the pediatrician.
    4. call the poison control center.

41. A restraint that may be used to prevent an adult patient from pulling on and removing tubes or an IV is a(n):
    1. vest restraint.
    2. jacket restraint.
    3. extremity restraint.
    4. mummy restraint.

42. An older adult patient in the extended care facility has been wandering outside of the room during the late evening hours. The patient has a history of falls. The nurse intervenes initially by:
    1. placing an abdominal restraint on the patient during the night.
    2. keeping both the light and the television on in the patient's room all night.
    3. reassigning the patient to a room close to the nursing station.
    4. having the family members check on the patient during the night.

43. A parent with three children has gone to the outpatient clinic. The children range in age from 2½ to 15 years old. A nurse is discussing safety issues with the parent. The nurse evaluates that further teaching is required if the parent states:
    1. "I have spoken to my teenager about safe sex practices."
    2. "I make sure that my child wears a helmet when he rides his bicycle."
    3. "My 8-year-old is taking swimming classes at the local community center."
    4. "Now my 2½-year-old can finally sit in the front seat of the car with me."

44. Bacteria that are spread through inadequate preparation or storage of food are:
    1. *Streptococcus*
    2. *Candida*
    3. *Listeria*
    4. *Hepatitis B*

STUDY GROUP QUESTIONS

- What are the basic human needs regarding safety?
- What are some physical hazards and how can they be reduced or eliminated?
- What developmental changes and abilities predispose individuals to accidents or injury?
- What additional risk factors may affect an individual's level of safety?
- What risks exist in a health care agency, and how can they be prevented?
- What safety measures and patient teaching should be implemented in different health care settings?
- What are the procedures for the correct use of side rails and restraints?
- How can a nurse avoid the use of patient restraints?
- What assessment information should be obtained regarding patient/family safety?
- How can a nurse assist patients and families in reducing or eliminating safety hazards?

STUDY CHART

- Create a chart to compare the specific safety issues for each developmental level.
- Assess your own home to determine if there are safety hazards that should be corrected.

Copyright © 2019, Elsevier Inc. All Rights Reserved.

31 Hygiene

PRELIMINARY READING

Chapter 31, pp. 812–864

CASE STUDIES

1. Your clinical experience is scheduled to be on a medical unit. It will be your responsibility to provide instruction to a patient who has just been diagnosed with diabetes mellitus.
   a. What specific information on hygienic care will be included for the patient's teaching session?

2. An older adult patient residing in an extended care facility requires assistance with hygienic care.
   a. What developmental changes are considered when assisting this patient to meet hygienic needs?

3. The student asks the primary nurse on the unit why he is giving the patient's bath and not just having the nurse's aide do it.
   a. How should the nurse respond?

CHAPTER REVIEW

Match the description/definition in Column A with the correct term in Column B.

	Column A	Column B
_____	1. Long, light gliding strokes used in massage	a. Abrasion
_____	2. Painful inflammation of oral mucous membranes	b. Edentulous
_____	3. Inflammation of the tissue surrounding the nail	c. Plantar wart
_____	4. Scraping or rubbing away of the epidermis, resulting in localized bleeding	d. Perineal care
_____	5. Keratosis caused by friction and pressure from shoes, mainly on toes	e. Contact dermatitis
_____	6. Fungating lesion that appears on the sole of the foot	f. Corn
_____	7. Loss of hair	g. Gingivitis
_____	8. Without teeth	h. Paronychia
_____	9. Abnormal dryness of the skin	i. Callus
_____	10. Cleansing of the patients' genital and anal areas	j. Alopecia
_____	11. Inflammation of the skin characterized by abrupt onset with erythema, pruritus, pain, and scaly oozing lesions	k. Maceration
_____	12. Thickened portion of the epidermis, usually flat and painless, on the undersurface of the foot or hand	l. Effleurage
_____	13. Softening	m. Mucositis
_____	14. Inflammation of the gums	n. Xerosis

Copyright © 2019, Elsevier Inc. All Rights Reserved.

Complete the following:

15. Identify at least three factors that contribute to *Inability to perform self care: hygiene.*

16. What modifications are done when providing hygienic care to a patient with dementia?

17. Which of the following techniques are appropriate for diabetic foot care? Select all that apply.

    a. Soaking the feet _____

    b. Rubbing the feet vigorously to dry them _____

    c. Walking barefoot to toughen the feet _____

    d. Applying extra lotion between the toes _____

    e. Wearing clean, white cotton socks _____

    f. Using a heating pad to warm the feet _____

    g. Applying a mild antiseptic to small cuts _____

    h. Avoiding elastic stockings _____

18. A nurse-initiated treatment for a skin rash is:

19. When cleansing a patient's eyes, the nurse should use:

20. The nurse recognizes that the skin goes through changes throughout the life span. Which of the following are accurate statements regarding the characteristics of the skin? Select all that apply.

    a. Neonatal skin is thinner. _____

    b. The sebaceous glands become active during the toddler years. _____

    c. Young adult skin should be elastic, firm, and smooth. _____

    d. The sweat glands are fully functional at puberty. _____

    e. Skin thickens progressively with aging. _____

    f. Lubrication from the skin glands diminishes over time. _____

21. For hygienic care, the nurse applies the ethical principle of autonomy, which means that the nurse should: _____

    _____.

22. When is a standing shower contraindicated for a patient?

23. For the patient with a nursing diagnosis of *Unable to tolerate activity*, how can hygienic care be affected?

24. Identify ways that the nurse can promote healthy skin for the patient.

25. a. Cotton-tipped applicators should be used to remove ear wax.

    True _____ False _____

    b. A 5–10 minute bath can add moisture to the skin of an older adult.

    True _____ False _____

26. The nurse wants to help the patient to have healthy teeth and gums. Which of the following recommendations should be made to the patient? Select all that apply.

    a. Change the toothbrush every 6–8 months. _____

    b. Use a soft bristle toothbrush with a straight handle. _____

    c. Floss at least once each day. _____

    d. Brush the teeth at least once each day. _____

    e. Use a toothbrush cover to protect the bristles.

    _____

27. Evidence-based practice indicates that this product is more effective than soap in reducing the bacteria found in wash basins: _____

    _____.

28. Care of the patient's eyeglasses includes:

Copyright © 2019, Elsevier Inc. All Rights Reserved.

29. Ear irrigation is contraindicated in the presence of:

30. Asepsis is maintained during linen changes when the nurse:

31. Provide an example of how the nurse prepares a comfortable environment for the patient in the health care facility:

32. Identify physiological conditions that may place a patient at risk for impaired skin integrity.

33. How does the use of a commercial "bag bath" differ from a regular patient bed bath?

34. Identify a safety measure that is implemented when providing a tub bath for a patient.

35. How may patients' cultural backgrounds influence their hygienic care practices?

36. A nurse notes that a young adult patient has acne of the face and back. What care should be provided?

37. Identify at least three guidelines for patient bathing and skin care.

38. What patients may require special oral hygiene?

39. Place the steps of the bed bath in the correct order:

a. Back _____

b. Arms _____

c. Face _____

d. Abdomen _____

e. Legs _____

f. Perineal area _____

g. Chest _____

40. Identify safety measures that should be implemented during oral care for an unconscious patient.

41. What is the procedure for irrigation of the ear?

42. Prior to providing nail care for a patient who is not diabetic, the nurse should:

43. During the bath, the nurse assesses the patient carefully. There are signs of vascular insufficiency in the lower extremities. This is determined based upon finding:

44. Normal oral mucosa appears:

45. For the patient who uses a hearing aid, which are the appropriate instructions for the nurse to provide to the patient? Select all that apply.

a. Check for whistling sounds. _____

b. Wear the hearing aid continuously. _____

c. Store the hearing aid in a warm, heated place.

_____

d. Use alcohol to clean the hearing aid. _____

e. Have the patient check the battery while the hearing aid is in the ear. _____

f. Remove the battery if the hearing aid is not going to be used for a day or two. _____

131

Copyright © 2019, Elsevier Inc. All Rights Reserved.

46. a. Identify factors that affect the older adult's ability to manage foot care.

b. What common foot problems do older adults experience?

47. The patient is sitting up in a shower chair and tells you that he feels lightheaded and weak. What do you do?

48. What areas require special consideration during a skin assessment?

49. To protect yourself against infestation, what precautions are needed to a patient with pediculosis capitis?

50. For a patient on chemotherapy with injured oral mucosa, what special care should be provided?

51. A nurse is caring for an older adult patient in an extended care facility. The patient wears dentures, and the nurse delegated their care to the nursing assistant. The nurse instructs the assistant that the patient's dentures should be: Select all that apply.

a. Cleaned in hot water. _____

b. Left in place during the night. _____

c. Brushed with a soft toothbrush. _____

d. Wrapped in a soft towel when not worn. _____

e. Removed and rinsed after eating. _____

f. Rinsed in the sink lined with a towel. _____

52. Regardless of the type of bath being given, the nurse should use what guidelines?

53. a. Permission is needed to cut or braid a patient's hair.

True _____ False _____

b. A health care provider's order is always needed to do shampoos for patients.

Tue _____ False _____

c. It is not necessary to explain hygiene care procedures being done to patients who are unconscious.

True _____ False _____

54. Skin tears can occur in older adults. To reduce the risk of skin tears, you should:

55. Which of the following techniques are correct for bed making? Select all that apply.
a. Keep the sheets clean, dry, and free of wrinkles.

_____

b. Hold the linen close to your body after removing from the bed. _____

c. Never shake linen. _____

d. Place soiled linen on the floor. _____

e. Always raise the bed to the appropriate height before changing linen. _____

f. Return the bed to its lowest horizontal position after finishing. _____

g. Avoid bringing excess linen into the patient's room. _____

h. When a patient is discharged, send all bed linen to the laundry. _____

56. What are the techniques for female and male perineal care?

57. Provide the description and uses for the following bed positions:
a. Fowler's

b. Trendelenburg

Copyright © 2019, Elsevier Inc. All Rights Reserved.

58. Indicate the signs of peripheral neuropathy. Select all that apply.

   a. Decreased hair growth on legs and feet _____

   b. Foot deformities _____

   c. Shiny appearance of the skin _____

   d. Abnormal gait _____

   e. Thickened nails _____

   f. Decreased or absent vibratory, touch, temperature, or painful stimuli _____

Select the best answer for each of the following questions:

59. A nurse is caring for an older adult patient in an extended care facility. The patient wears dentures, and the nurse delegated their care to the nursing assistant. The nurse instructs the assistant that the patient's dentures should be:
   1. cleaned in hot water.
   2. left in place during the night.
   3. brushed with a soft toothbrush.
   4. wrapped in a soft towel when not worn.

60. A nurse determines, after completing an assessment, that an expected outcome for a patient with the potential for altered skin integrity will be that the skin:
   1. remains dry and intact.
   2. has increased erythema.
   3. tingles in areas of pressure.
   4. demonstrates increased diaphoresis.

61. A patient has been hospitalized following a traumatic injury. The nurse is now able to provide hair care for the patient. The nurse includes:
   1. using hot water to rinse the scalp.
   2. cutting away matted or tangled hair.
   3. using the fingernails to massage the patient's scalp.
   4. applying peroxide to dissolve blood in the hair and then rinsing with saline.

62. While completing a patient's bath, a nurse notices a red, raised skin rash on the patient's chest. The next step for the nurse to take is to:
   1. moisturize the skin with lotion.
   2. wash the area again with hot water and soap.
   3. discuss proper hygienic care with the patient.
   4. assess for any other areas of inflammation.

63. A nurse is planning patient assignment with a nursing assistant. In delegating the morning care for a patient, the nurse expects the assistant to:
   1. cut the patient's nails with scissors.
   2. use soap to wash the patient's eyes.
   3. wash the patient's legs with long strokes from the ankle to the knee.
   4. place the unconscious patient in high Fowler's position to provide oral hygiene.

64. A patient is receiving chemotherapy and is experiencing stomatitis. To promote comfort for this patient, a nurse recommends that the patient use:
   1. a firm toothbrush.
   2. normal saline rinses.
   3. a commercial mouthwash.
   4. an alcohol and water mixture.

65. For a patient with dry skin, a nurse should:
   1. apply moisturizing lotion.
   2. use hot water for bathing.
   3. obtain a dehumidifier.
   4. decrease fluid intake.

66. Use of an electric razor is specifically indicated for a patient who is being treated with:
   1. diuretics.
   2. antibiotics.
   3. anticoagulants.
   4. narcotic analgesics.

67. When making an occupied bed, the first step for a nurse is to:
   1. cover the patient with a bath blanket.
   2. explain the procedure to the patient.
   3. position the patient on the far side of the bed.
   4. adjust the height of the bed to waist level.

68. The nurse is providing information to a group of parents. Which of the following statements provides accurate information about the teeth?
   1. Permanent teeth are in place at 13 years of age.
   2. Wisdom teeth erupt in the 35 and older age group.
   3. The first permanent teeth come in at around 3 years of age.
   4. Teething occurs after the child reaches 2 years old.

69. The nurse manager is evaluating a new staff member's patient care. Which of the following interventions demonstrates correct technique?
   1. Placing the bedpan on the overbed table
   2. Returning extra linens from the patient's room to the linen cart
   3. Using side rails all the time to keep the patient safely in bed
   4. Raising the bed up to change the linen and reposition the patient

70. The individual's skin becomes more resistant to injury and infection, with the layers being more tightly bound together during which developmental stage?
   1. Infant
   2. Toddler
   3. School age
   4. Adolescent

Copyright © 2019, Elsevier Inc. All Rights Reserved.

STUDY GROUP QUESTIONS

- What hygienic care measures are necessary for the integumentary system?
- What factors may influence a patient's hygiene care practices?
- How do growth and development influence hygiene care needs?
- What are the patient teaching needs for hygiene care across the life span?
- What assessments of the integumentary system are necessary to determine alterations and hygiene care needs?
- What are the correct procedures for providing hygiene care and a comfortable environment for patients?

- What are the general safety guidelines for providing hygiene care?
- How does a patient's self-care ability influence the provision of hygiene care?
- How is physical assessment integrated into the provision of hygiene care?
- What actions should be taken if a patient refuses or is agitated during hygiene care?
- How is hygiene care altered for patients who are unconscious and/or unable to assist with care?
- Which hygiene care measures are appropriate to delegate?
- What equipment and supplies are needed to provide hygiene and maintain a comfortable environment for patients?

Copyright © 2019, Elsevier Inc. All Rights Reserved.

32 Oxygenation

PRELIMINARY READING

Chapter 32, pp. 865–916

CASE STUDIES

1. You are the nurse in an outpatient clinic where a 32-year-old woman has gone for ongoing medical treatment. She tells you that she has had asthma since she was a young child. While speaking with the patient, you notice that she is exhibiting mild wheezing and a productive cough. She appears slightly pale.
   a. What additional assessment questions should be asked of this patient?
   b. Identify a possible nursing diagnosis for this patient.
   c. What nurse-initiated actions may be taken at this time?
   d. Identify general information that should be included in patient teaching for promoting oxygenation.

2. The patient had thoracic surgery yesterday afternoon and has a chest tube in place. You are checking the drainage and note that there is a sudden increase in the amount and it is definitely bloody.
   a. What should you do?
   b. What could be causing this increase in drainage?

CHAPTER REVIEW

Match the description/definition in Column A with the correct term in Column B.

Column A	Column B
_____ 1. Collapse of alveoli, preventing exchange of oxygen	a. Hypoxia
_____ 2. Tachypnea pattern of breathing associated with metabolic acidosis	b. Pneumothorax
_____ 3. Need to sit upright to breathe easier	c. Atelectasis
_____ 4. Collection of air in the pleural space	d. Kussmaul respiration
_____ 5. Bloody sputum	e. Orthopnea
_____ 6. Inadequate tissue oxygenation	f. Hemothorax
_____ 7. Amount of blood in the ventricles at the end of diastole	g. Preload
_____ 8. Collection of blood in the pleural space	h. Afterload
_____ 9. Resistance of ejection of blood from the left ventricle	i. Hemoptysis
_____ 10. Difficulty breathing, sensation of breathlessness	j. Dyspnea

Copyright © 2019, Elsevier Inc. All Rights Reserved.

Complete the following:

11. The average heart rate for an adult is between ___–___ beats per minute.

12. Chest movement is affected by what conditions?

13. Identify whether the following signs and symptoms are associated with left ventricular or right ventricular heart failure:

    a. Dyspnea _____

    b. Distended neck veins _____

    c. Ankle edema _____

    d. Pulmonary congestion _____

14. Which of the following may cause hyperventilation? Select all that apply.

    a. Anxiety _____

    b. Fever _____

    c. Severe atelectasis _____

    d. Head injury _____

    e. Excessive administration of oxygen _____

15. Provide an example of a physiological alteration or problem that may cause each of the following:
    a. Decreased oxygen carrying capacity
    b. Decreased inspired oxygen concentration
    c. Hypovolemia
    d. Increased metabolic rate

16. A premature infant has a deficiency of _____ and is at risk for hyaline membrane disease.

17. An example of a controllable risk factor for cardiopulmonary disease is:

18. Which of the following pathophysiological changes in the heart and lungs occur with aging? Select all that apply.
    a. Thinning of the ventricular wall of the heart _____

    b. SA node becoming fibrotic from calcification _____

    c. Increased elastin in the arterial vessel walls _____

    d. Increased chest wall compliance and elastic recoil _____

    e. Decreased alveolar surface area _____

    f. Increased responsiveness of central and peripheral chemoreceptors _____

    g. Decreased number of cilia _____

    h. Increased respiratory drive _____

19. A patient awakens in a panic and feels as though she is suffocating. This is noted by the nurse as:

20. A musical, high-pitched lung sound that may be heard on inspiration or expiration is:

21. Identify what should be done if the hospitalized patient's monitor is showing ventricular fibrillation.

22. Briefly define the following abnormal chest wall movements:
    a. Retraction
    b. Paradoxical breathing

23. Which type of asepsis is used for tracheal suctioning?

24. Continuous bubbling in the chest tube water-seal chamber indicates:

25. Identify an example of a nursing intervention for promotion of each of the following:
    a. Dyspnea management
    b. Patent airway
    c. Lung expansion
    d. Mobilization of secretions

Copyright © 2019, Elsevier Inc. All Rights Reserved.

26. Identify the following types of oxygen delivery systems and the flow rate for each:

a.

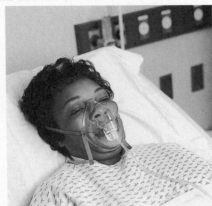

b.

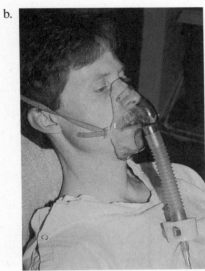

27. Identify the following for tuberculin (Mantoux) testing:
   a. A skin test is administered on a patient's:

   b. The test is read after _____ hours.

   c. A reddened, flat area is a(n) _____ reaction.

   d. The patient received a Bacille Calmette-Guerin (BCG) vaccination, so the tuberculin skin test will most likely be:

   Positive _____ Negative _____

28. For chest percussion, vibration, and postural drainage:
   a. Chest percussion is contraindicated for a patient with:

   b. Chest percussion may be done over multiple layers of clothing.

   True _____ False _____

   c. Vibration is used only during:

   d. Briefly explain high-frequency chest wall compression (HFCWC) and identify the patients who may benefit most from its use.

29. For continuous positive airway pressure (CPAP):
   a. CPAP is used for:
   b. The usual pressure setting is:
   c. A disadvantage of CPAP is:
   d. How is BiPAP different from CPAP?

30. For home oxygen therapy:
   a. It is indicated when the patient has a SaO_2 value of:
   b. What safety measures should be implemented when oxygen is used in the home?

31. The interventions in CPR are:
   C -
   A -
   B -

   The rate of chest compressions for an adult is _____ /minute.

32. Defibrillation is recommended within _____ (time) for an out-of-hospital sudden cardiac arrest and within _____ (time) for an inpatient.

33. a. The prevalence of atrial fibrillation increases with age.

   True _____ False _____
   b. Care of chest tubes can be delegated to a nursing assistant.

   True _____ False _____

34. The patient has oxygen via a nasal cannula. What specific nursing care should be provided for this patient?

35. For the nursing diagnosis *Insufficient airway clearance related to the presence of tracheobronchial secretions*, identify a patient outcome and a nursing intervention to assist the patient to meet the outcome.

36. Which of the following are appropriate interventions for patient suctioning? Select all that apply.
   a. Performing pharyngeal suctioning before tracheal suctioning _____

   b. Avoiding routine use of normal saline instillations when suctioning _____

   c. Applying suction for 30 seconds at a time _____

   d. Suctioning during the insertion and removal of the tube _____

   e. Allowing 1–2 minutes between suction passes _____

   f. Providing regular suctioning every 1–2 hours around the clock _____

137

Copyright © 2019, Elsevier Inc. All Rights Reserved.

37. Cardiac output is the result of the stroke volume × _____.

38. For a patient with hypoxia:
    a. What are the signs and symptoms?
    b. What treatment is anticipated?

39. Identify a possible nursing diagnosis for a patient with anemia.

40. Provide examples of dietary risks that may influence cardiopulmonary status and oxygenation.

41. The most effective positioning for a patient with cardiopulmonary disease is:

42. A method to encourage voluntary deep breathing for a postoperative patient is the use of a(n):

43. Identify at least two environmental or occupational hazards that may affect an individual's cardiopulmonary functioning:

44. Cardiac dysrhythmias may be caused by:

45. The nurse anticipates that atrial fibrillation will be treated with:

46. In order to reduce the incidence of ventilator associated pneumonia (VAP), the nurse will implement:

47. The nurse anticipates that treatment for hyperventilation will include:

48. Place the following steps for in-line suctioning in the correct sequence. The nurse has already positioned the patient and performed hand hygiene.
    a. Reassess pulmonary status _____
    b. Insert the catheter until resistance is felt _____
    c. Hyperoxygenate the patient _____
    d. Withdraw the catheter, applying suction _____
    e. Repeat the procedure, if indicated _____
    f. Pick up the catheter enclosed in the plastic sheath _____

49. Identify the areas on the chest tube system.

50. Identify the appropriate care for a patient with a closed chest tube drainage system in place. Select all that apply.
    a. Clamp the chest tube when the patient ambulates. _____
    b. Milk the tube for the patient who has just had thoracic surgery, if necessary. _____
    c. Instruct the patient to inhale if the tube disconnects. _____
    d. Report over 100 mL of sanguinous drainage after the patient is more than 8 hours postoperative.
    e. Keep the drainage unit upright. _____

51. Identify at least three pathologies that reduce chest wall expansion.

Copyright © 2019, Elsevier Inc. All Rights Reserved.

52. Signs and symptoms of cardiac pain in women include:

53. What factors contribute to respiratory problems in infants and young children?

54. Which of the following are lifestyle factors that contribute to poor cardiopulmonary status? Select all that apply.

    a. Having a diet low in protein _____

    b. Participating in a daily exercise regimen _____

    c. Drinking significant amounts of alcohol _____

    d. Being a construction worker _____

    e. Having a high stress job _____

55. An early sign that the patient's chronic cardiopulmonary disease is worsening is: _____.

56. The patient becomes breathless and tired during the physical exam. The nurse should:

57. Nebulization is used in the administration of what types of medications?

58. A Yankauer suction catheter is used for _____ _____ suction.

59. Positioning for the patient with right-sided atelectasis will be on the left or right side?

60. What medication is contraindicated for a patient with asthma?

61. Caution is used when administering oxygen to patients with chronic lung disease because:

62. Individuals have gone to the health fair to receive their free influenza vaccine. The nurse briefly discusses the medical backgrounds of the patients. The influenza vaccine will be withheld from the following individuals: Select all that apply.

    a. Three-month-old child _____

    b. Older adult woman _____

    c. Man with chronic arthritis _____

    d. Woman with a severe hypersensitivity to eggs _____

    e. A woman with a history of Guillain-Barré syndrome _____

63. How is oxygenation affected in the individual who is receiving chemotherapy?

64. a. Identify at least four signs or symptoms of hypoventilation.
    b. How is hypoventilation treated?

65. Identify the signs/symptoms of dyspnea. Select all that apply.

    a. Labored breathing _____

    b. Nasal flaring _____

    c. Chest pain _____

    d. Increased respiratory rate _____

    e. Coughing _____

66. Indicate at least three examples of health education in the community for prevention or identification of cardiopulmonary disease.

67. Which of the following herbs or spices are contraindicated for patients with high blood pressure or asthma? Select all that apply.

    a. Pepper _____

    b. Ginseng _____

    c. Paprika _____

    d. Ma huang _____

    e. Garlic capsules _____

68. What personal protective equipment (PPE) is used when preparing to suction a patient?

Copyright © 2019, Elsevier Inc. All Rights Reserved.

69. After suctioning, the patient has a decrease in overall cardiopulmonary status as evidenced by decreased SpO_2, increased $EtCO_2$, continued tachypnea, continued straining to breathe, bronchospasm, and cardiac dysrhythmia. What should the nurse do?

70. Focused assessment of a patient's breathing pattern includes:

Select the best answer for each of the following questions:

71. A patient has a chest tube in place to drain bloody secretions from the chest cavity. When caring for a patient with a chest tube, a nurse should:
    1. keep the drainage device above chest level.
    2. clamp the chest tube when the patient is ambulating.
    3. apply an occlusive dressing if the tubing becomes dislodged.
    4. leave trapped fluid in the tubing and estimate the amount.

72. A nurse is making a home visit to a patient who has emphysema (chronic obstructive pulmonary disease [COPD]). Specific instruction to control exhalation pressure for this patient with an increased residual volume of air should include:
    1. coughing.
    2. deep breathing.
    3. pursed-lip breathing.
    4. diaphragmatic breathing.

73. A patient has been admitted to a medical center with a respiratory condition and dyspnea. A number of medications are prescribed for the patient. For a patient with this difficulty, the nurse should question the order for:
    1. steroids.
    2. mucolytics.
    3. bronchodilators.
    4. narcotic analgesics.

74. After a patient assessment, the nurse suspects hypoxemia. This is based on the nurse finding that the patient is experiencing:
    1. restlessness.
    2. bradypnea.
    3. bradycardia.
    4. hypotension.

75. A patient has experienced some respiratory difficulty and is placed on oxygen via nasal cannula. A nurse assists the patient with this form of oxygen delivery by:
    1. changing the tubing every 4 hours.
    2. assessing the nares for breakdown.
    3. inspecting the back of the mouth q8h.
    4. securing the cannula to the nose with nonallergic tape.

76. A patient is being seen in an outpatient medical clinic. A nurse has reviewed the patient's chart and finds that there is a history of a cardiopulmonary abnormality. This is supported by the nurse's assessment of the patient having:
    1. scleral jaundice.
    2. reddened conjunctivae.
    3. symmetrical chest movement.
    4. clubbing of the fingertips.

77. A 65-year-old patient is seen in a physician's office for a routine annual checkup. As part of the physical examination, an ECG is performed. The ECG reveals a normal P wave, P-R interval, and QRS complex and a heart rate of 58 beats per minute. The nurse evaluates this finding as:
    1. sinus tachycardia.
    2. sinus bradycardia.
    3. sinus dysrhythmia.
    4. supraventricular bradycardia.

78. A patient is admitted to a medical center with a diagnosis of left ventricular congestive heart failure. A nurse is completing the physical assessment and is anticipating finding that the patient has:
    1. liver enlargement.
    2. peripheral edema.
    3. pulmonary congestion.
    4. jugular neck vein distention.

79. A patient has just returned to the unit after abdominal surgery. A nurse is planning care for this patient and is considering interventions to specifically promote pulmonary function and prevent complications. The nurse first:
    1. teaches the patient leg exercises to perform.
    2. asks the physician to order nebulizer treatments.
    3. demonstrates the use of a flow-oriented incentive spirometer.
    4. informs the patient that his secretions will need to be suctioned.

80. A nurse manager is evaluating the care that is provided by a new staff nurse during the orientation period. One of the patients requires nasotracheal suctioning, and the nurse manager determines that the appropriate technique is used when the new staff nurse:
    1. places the patient in the supine position.
    2. prepares for a clean or nonsterile procedure.
    3. suctions the oropharyngeal area first, then moves to the nasotracheal area.
    4. applies intermittent suction for 10 seconds while the suction catheter is being removed.

Copyright © 2019, Elsevier Inc. All Rights Reserved.

81. Chest tubes have been inserted into a patient after thoracic surgery. In working with this patient, a nurse should:
    1. coil and secure excess tubing next to the patient.
    2. clamp off the chest tubes except during respiratory assessments.
    3. milk or strip the tubing every 15–30 minutes to maintain drainage.
    4. remove the tubing from the connection to check for adequate suction.

82. A patient is being discharged home with an order for oxygen PRN. In preparing to teach the patient and family, a priority for the nurse is to provide information on the:
    1. use of the oxygen delivery equipment.
    2. physiology of the respiratory system.
    3. use of PaO_2 levels to determine oxygen demand.
    4. length of time that the oxygen is to be used by the patient.

83. In discriminating types of chest pain that a patient may experience, a nurse recognizes that pain associated with inflammation of the pericardial sac is noted by the patient experiencing:
    1. knife-like pain to the upper chest.
    2. constant, substernal pain.
    3. pain with inspiration.
    4. pain aggravated by coughing.

84. A nurse is checking a patient who has a chest tube in place and finds that there is constant bubbling in the water-seal chamber. The nurse should:
    1. secure any loose connections.
    2. leave the chest tube clamped.
    3. raise the tubing above the level of the insertion site.
    4. prepare the patient for the removal of the tube.

85. The patient is admitted with a diagnosis of COPD. The appropriate oxygen delivery method for this patient is a:
    1. simple face mask with 5–8 L/min (50%) O_2.
    2. Venturi mask with 8 L/min (35%–40%) O_2.
    3. nasal cannula with 1–2 L/min (28%) O_2.
    4. partial nonrebreather mask with 6–10 L/min (80%) O_2.

86. A nurse is completing a physical assessment of a patient with a history of a cardiopulmonary abnormality. A finding associated with hyperlipidemia is the patient having:
    1. cyanosis.
    2. xanthelasma.
    3. petechiae.
    4. ecchymosis.

87. During patient assessment, which of the following is an expected sign of hypoxemia?
    1. Pale conjunctivae
    2. Central cyanosis
    3. Dependent edema
    4. Splinter hemorrhages

88. For postural drainage for the lower lobes, the patient is best placed in which position?
    1. Trendelenburg
    2. Prone, horizontal
    3. High Fowler's
    4. Three-fourths supine

89. For patients at risk of or having cardiopulmonary issues, the target blood pressure for people below 60 years of age is less than:
    1. 110/70
    2. 120/80
    3. 140/90
    4. 150/80

90. The nurse documents the patient's periods of increasing depths of breathing, followed by period of apnea, as:
    1. eupnea.
    2. bradypnea.
    3. ataxic.
    4. Cheyne-Stokes.

STUDY GROUP QUESTIONS

- How do the anatomy and physiology of the cardiovascular and respiratory systems promote oxygenation?
- What physiological factors affect oxygenation?
- How do growth and development influence oxygenation?
- How do behavioral and environmental factors influence oxygenation?
- What are some common alterations in cardiovascular and pulmonary functioning?
- How are the critical thinking and nursing processes applied to patients having difficulty with oxygenation?
- What assessment information should be obtained to determine the patient's oxygenation status?
- What findings are usually seen in a patient who has inadequate oxygenation?
- How can the nurse promote oxygenation for patients in the health promotion, acute care, and restorative care settings?
- What specific measures and procedures should be implemented by the nurse to manage dyspnea, maintain a patent airway, mobilize secretions, and expand the lungs?
- What should be included in patient/family teaching for promotion and maintenance of oxygenation?
- What safety measures should be implemented for the use of oxygen in the home?

Copyright © 2019, Elsevier Inc. All Rights Reserved.

33 Sleep

PRELIMINARY READING

Chapter 33, pp. 917–938

CASE STUDIES

1. A middle-aged adult patient has gone to a physician's office to obtain a prescription for a "sleeping pill" because she has been having difficulty either falling or staying asleep. You are completing the initial nursing assessment and discover that the patient is recently divorced and trying to juggle extensive work and child care responsibilities.
   a. Identify a possible nursing diagnosis and outcome for this patient.
   b. Indicate nursing interventions and teaching areas for this patient.

2. A nurse has just been moved to the night shift in the hospital and starts to experience difficulty in getting to sleep when he gets home. He is finding it harder to focus at work.
   a. What can be done to assist the nurse in adapting to the change in his work schedule and sleep pattern?

3. You visit the home of a patient who was recently discharged from the hospital. The patient tells you that she needs to get up several times during the night to go to the bathroom. You observe that she has laundry baskets in the hallway, minimal lighting in the hallway, tile floors in the bathroom, and a hamper in the bedroom.
   a. What are your concerns for this patient?
   b. What can you instruct the patient to do to help reduce the number of times she gets up?

CHAPTER REVIEW

Match the description/definition in Column A with the correct term in Column B.

Column A	Column B
_____ 1. Cessation of breathing for periods of time during sleep	a. Cataplexy
_____ 2. A decrease in the amount, quality, and consistency of sleep	b. Sleep deprivation
_____ 3. Awaking at night to urinate	c. Circadian rhythm
_____ 4. Sudden muscle weakness during intense emotions	d. Parasomnia
_____ 5. Difficulty falling or staying asleep	e. Sleep
_____ 6. 24-hour day/night cycle	f. Sleep apnea
_____ 7. Sleep disorders that can occur during arousal from REM or partial arousal from NREM sleep	g. Insomnia
_____ 8. Excessive sleepiness during the day	h. Nocturia
_____ 9. A recurrent, altered state of consciousness that occurs for sustained periods	i. Narcolepsy

Copyright © 2019, Elsevier Inc. All Rights Reserved.

Complete the following:

10. Provide examples of factors that may affect sleep.

11. Which of the following are appropriate nursing interventions to assist the older adult patient to achieve adequate sleep? Select all that apply.

    a. Altering the daily sleep and wake times _____

    b. Encouraging the patient to stay in bed even if not feeling sleepy _____

    c. Limiting patient's caffeine intake in the late afternoon or evening _____

    d. Lowering the head of the bed as flat as possible _____

    e. Encouraging increased fluid intake 2–4 hours before sleep _____

    f. Avoiding use of sedatives and hypnotics, if possible _____

    g. Encouraging daytime naps of 1–2 hours _____

    h. Provide social activities and exercise _____

12. Identify a way in which a nurse can promote a restful environment in the acute care setting.

13. It is expected that during sleep the heart rate will decrease by about 10 beats per minute from the daytime average rate.

    True _____ False _____

14. Very few older adults experience sleep problems.

    True _____ False _____

15. Normal sleep cycles usually last _____ (time) and are followed by _____ sleep.

16. Identify at least two nursing interventions that may be implemented related to a patient's sleep:
    a. Comfort measures
    b. Safety measures

17. A nurse tells a patient to include what information in a sleep diary?

18. a. What are the best types of bedtime snacks for promoting sleep?

    b. A nutritional supplement that may be used to promote sleep is _____ at a dosage of _____ mg two hours before bedtime.

19. A nurse recommends to the parents of a newborn that the best way to position the child for sleep is on his/her:

20. Identify at least one patient outcome related to sleep.

21. For sleep disturbances:
    a. What physical and behavioral problems may occur when individuals have an insufficient amount of sleep?
    b. What are the safety considerations for patients with narcolepsy, EDS, sleep deprivation, and/or nocturia?

22. Use of technology, such as cell phones, close to bedtime can lead to changes in sleep and excessive daytime sleepiness.

    True _____ False _____

23. What is the value of REM sleep?

24. a. Symptoms of obstructive sleep apnea (OSA) include:
    b. Central sleep apnea is frequently seen in patients who have which pathological conditions?

25. Identify at least two questions to ask in order to assess a patient's sleep habits.

26. For a patient with chronic insomnia, the nurse should:

27. For the patient with obstructive sleep apnea, identify the recommendations for health promotion. Select all that apply.

    a. Weight loss _____

    b. Use of benzodiazepines _____

    c. Change of bedtime routine _____

    d. Use of analgesics _____

    e. Elevating the head of the bed _____

143

Copyright © 2019, Elsevier Inc. All Rights Reserved.

28. Identify which of the following are nonbenzodiazepine, benzodiazepine receptor agonists. Select all that apply.

a. Flurazepam _____

b. Melatonin _____

c. Zolpidem _____

d. Triazolam _____

e. Eszopiclone _____

f. Zaleplon _____

29. Identify at least four measures to implement to improve the patient's comfort for sleep.

30. In long term care, one of the most important interventions to improve night time sleep is to _____.

31. Identify an effective, subjective method for assessing sleep quality.

32. After completing the STOP-BANG Questionnaire, the patient's score is 6 "Yes" responses. This indicates a _____ risk for Obstructive Sleep Apnea (OSA).

33. Current estimates show that 50–70 million adults in the United States have some type of sleep-wake problem.

True _____ False _____

Select the best answer for each of the following questions:

34. Individuals experience changes in their sleep patterns as they progress through the life cycle. A nurse assesses that a patient is experiencing bedtime fears, waking during the night, and nightmares. These behaviors are associated with:
1. infants.
2. toddlers.
3. preschoolers.
4. school-age children.

35. A nurse is making rounds during the night to check on patients. When she enters one of the rooms at 3:00 a.m., she finds that the patient is sitting up in a chair. The patient tells the nurse that she is not able to sleep. The nurse should first:
1. obtain an order for a hypnotic.
2. assist the patient back to bed.
3. provide a glass of warm milk and a back rub.
4. ask about activities that have previously helped her sleep.

36. A nurse is working on a pediatric unit at the local hospital. A 4-year-old boy is admitted to the unit. To assist this child to sleep, the nurse:
1. reads to him.
2. teaches him relaxation activities.
3. allows him to watch TV until he is tired.
4. has him get ready for bed very quickly, without advance notice.

37. A patient is found to be awakening frequently during the night. There are a number of medications prescribed for this patient. The nurse determines that the medication that may be creating this patient's particular sleep disturbance is the:
1. narcotic.
2. beta-adrenergic blocker.
3. antidepressant.
4. antihistamine.

38. A nurse suspects that a patient may be experiencing sleep deprivation. This suspicion is validated by the nurse's finding that the patient has:
1. increased reflex response.
2. blurred vision.
3. cardiac arrhythmias.
4. increased response time.

39. A nurse is working in a sleep clinic that is part of the local hospital. In preparing to work with patients with different sleep needs, the nurse understands that:
1. bedtime rituals are most important for adolescents.
2. regular use of sleeping medications is appropriate.
3. warm milk before bedtime may help a patient sleep.
4. individuals are most easily aroused from sleep during stages 3 and 4.

40. A nurse is visiting a patient in his home. While completing a patient history and home assessment, the nurse finds that there are many prescription medications kept in the bathroom cabinet. In determining possible areas that may influence the patient's sleep patterns, the nurse looks for a classification of medication that may suppress the patient's rapid eye movement (REM) sleep. The nurse looks in the cabinet specifically for a(n):
1. diuretic.
2. anticonvulsant.
3. benzodiazepine.
4. antihistamine.

Copyright © 2019, Elsevier Inc. All Rights Reserved.

41. A newborn is taken to a pediatrician's office for the first physical exam. The parents ask the nurse when they can expect the baby to sleep through the night. The nurse responds that, although there may be individual differences, infants usually develop a nighttime pattern of sleep by the age of:
    1. 6 weeks.
    2. 3 months.
    3. 6 months.
    4. 10 months.

42. A nurse is working with older adults in the senior center. A group is discussing problems with sleep. The nurse recognizes that older adults:
    1. take less time to fall asleep.
    2. are more difficult to arouse from sleep.
    3. have a significant decline in stage 4 sleep.
    4. require more sleep than a middle-aged adult.

43. A patient with congestive heart failure is being discharged from the hospital to her home. The patient will be taking a diuretic daily. The nurse recognizes that, with this drug, the patient may experience:
    1. nocturia.
    2. nightmares.
    3. reduced REM sleep.
    4. increased daytime sleepiness.

44. During a home visit, a nurse discovers that the patient has been having difficulty sleeping. To assist the patient to achieve sufficient sleep, an appropriate question the nurse might ask is the following:
    1. "Do you keep your bedroom completely dark at night?"
    2. "Do you nap enough during the day?"
    3. "Why don't you eat something right before you go to bed?"
    4. "What kinds of things do you do right before bedtime?"

45. A patient has gone to the sleep clinic to determine what may be creating his sleeping problems. In addition, his partner is having sleep pattern interruptions. If this patient is experiencing sleep apnea, the nurse may expect the partner to identify that the patient:
    1. snores excessively.
    2. talks in his sleep.
    3. is very restless.
    4. walks in his sleep.

46. A nurse anticipates that the patient who is in non–rapid eye movement (NREM) stage 1 sleep is:
    1. easily aroused.
    2. completely relaxed.
    3. having vivid, full-color dreams.
    4. experiencing significantly reduced vital signs.

47. A nurse is working with a patient who has a history of respiratory disease. This patient is expected to demonstrate a(n):
    1. longer time falling asleep.
    2. decreased NREM sleep.
    3. increased awakenings in the early morning.
    4. need for extra pillows for comfort.

48. To help promote sleep for a patient, a nurse recommends:
    1. exercise about 2 hours before bedtime.
    2. intake of a large meal about 3 hours before bedtime.
    3. drinking alcoholic beverages at bedtime.
    4. napping frequently during the afternoon.

49. An expected treatment for sleep apnea is:
    1. biofeedback.
    2. full body massage.
    3. administration of hypnotics.
    4. continuous positive airway pressure (CPAP).

50. As sleep aids, medications that are considered relatively safe to use are:
    1. nonbenzodiazepines.
    2. barbiturates.
    3. psychotropics.
    4. anticonvulsants.

51. An expected observation of a patient in REM sleep is:
    1. possible enuresis.
    2. sleepwalking.
    3. loss of skeletal muscle tone.
    4. easy arousal from external noise.

52. A parent asks the nurse what the appropriate amount of sleep is for her 11-year-old child. The nurse responds correctly by informing the parent that children in this age group should average:
    1. 14 hours per night.
    2. 12 hours per night.
    3. 10 hours per night.
    4. 7 hours per night.

53. Parents ask the nurse about having their child sleep in their bed with them. The nurse's best response is to:
    1. discourage the practice entirely.
    2. identify that the child will probably sleep more soundly with them.
    3. recommend that lots of soft bedding be used to protect the child.
    4. indicate that there are risks associated with this practice.

Copyright © 2019, Elsevier Inc. All Rights Reserved.

54. The patient uses CPAP at home and is admitted to the hospital for surgery. A priority assessment in the postoperative period is:
    1. oxygen saturation.
    2. CPAP functioning.
    3. sleep patterns.
    4. comfort level.

55. For the patient in NREM stage 4 sleep, which of the following is true?
    1. Muscles begin to become relaxed.
    2. The stage lasts about 10 minutes.
    3. Vital signs are significantly lower than during waking hours.
    4. If awakened, the person feels as though daydreaming has occurred.

56. Which of the following medications interferes with patients reaching deeper stages of sleep?
    1. Antidepressants
    2. Hypnotics
    3. Antihistamines
    4. Opiates

STUDY GROUP QUESTIONS

- What is sleep?
- What are the physiological processes involved in sleep?
- How is sleep regulated by the body?
- What are the functions of sleep?
- What purpose do dreams serve?
- What are the normal requirements and patterns of sleep across the life span?
- What factors may influence sleep?
- What are some common sleep disorders and nursing interventions?
- What information should be included in a sleep history?
- How are the critical thinking and nursing processes applied with patients experiencing insufficient sleep or rest?
- What measures may be implemented by the nurse to promote sleep for patients/families?
- What information should be included in patient/family teaching for the promotion of rest and sleep?

STUDY CHART

Create a study chart to describe the *Sleep Patterns Across the Life Span* that identifies the sleep patterns and needs for infants, toddlers, preschoolers, school-age children, adolescents, adults, and older adults.

Copyright © 2019, Elsevier Inc. All Rights Reserved.

34 Pain Management

PRELIMINARY READING

PRELIMINARY READING

Chapter 34, pp. 939–971

CASE STUDIES

1. A patient is going to be using a PCA pump with a morphine infusion after surgery.
   a. What assessments need to be made before and while the patient uses the pump?
   b. What medications are usually prescribed for PCA?
   c. What information is needed in the teaching plan for this patient?

2. You are admitting a patient who is in labor. She tells you that this is her second child and that she had a "hard time having the first one because the pain was just horrible."
   a. What are the possible expectations of this patient?
   b. In applying the QSEN competency of patient-centered care, what nursing interventions do you include for this patient?

CHAPTER REVIEW

Match the description/definition in Column A with the correct term in Column B.

	Column A	Column B
_____	1. Local anesthesia, with minimal sedation, given between the vertebrae	a. Pain
_____	2. Unpleasant, subjective sensory and emotional experience	b. Analgesic
_____	3. Sensation of pain distant from the actual site	c. Exacerbation
_____	4. Results from tissue injury	d. Referred pain
_____	5. Protective, rapid onset, lasts briefly	e. Acute pain
_____	6. Increase in the severity of symptoms	f. Chronic pain
_____	7. Classification of medication used for pain relief	g. Nociceptive pain
_____	8. Prolonged, varying in intensity	h. Epidural infusion

Complete the following:

9. Identify and briefly describe the four physiological processes of pain.

10. The gate control theory of pain suggests that pain can be reduced through the use of:

11. Which of the following are physiological responses to acute pain as a result of sympathetic stimulation? Select all that apply.

   a. Decreased respiratory rate _____

   b. Increased heart rate _____

   c. Peripheral vasodilation _____

   d. Increased blood glucose level _____

   e. Diaphoresis _____

   f. Pupil constriction _____

   g. Decreased blood pressure _____

147

Copyright © 2019, Elsevier Inc. All Rights Reserved.

12. For a patient with chronic pain, identify the following:
    a. Associated symptoms
    b. An example of a lifestyle response to chronic pain

13. a. Identify two responses that an infant or child could have to pain.
    b. Identify two responses that adults could have to acute pain.

14. The single most reliable indicator of pain is the:

15. Using the PQRSTU assessment guide, identify nursing interventions for the following.
    a. Quality
    b. Region
    c. Timing

16. Identify how a nurse may assess the level of pain for the following patients.
    a. Toddler

    b. Person for whom English is a second language

    c. Person with dementia

17. a. To determine the location of a patient's pain, a nurse should ask the patient to:
    b. The patient indicates that the discomfort is located in the right side of the abdomen. Provide an example of how the pain experience could be appropriately documented for this patient.

18. A pain rating of _____ on a scale of 0–10 is an emergency and requires immediate action.

19. For a patient who experiences discomfort upon ambulation or during a dressing change, a nurse should plan to:

20. An example of how a nurse may individualize a patient's treatment for pain is:

21. Which of the following are correct statements regarding transcutaneous electrical nerve stimulation (TENS)? Select all that apply.

    a. It is an invasive procedure. _____

    b. It requires a health care provider's order. _____

    c. Only a specially certified person can use the device. _____

    d. Electrodes are applied directly onto the skin. _____

    e. Controls are adjusted until the patient feels a tingling sensation. _____

22. Which of the following medications are indicated for the treatment of mild to moderate pain? Select all that apply.

    a. Ibuprofen _____

    b. Morphine _____

    c. Codeine _____

    d. Fentanyl _____

    e. Acetaminophen _____

    f. Hydromorphone _____

23. Identify two examples of nonpharmacological interventions that may be implemented to relieve pain.

24. An example of an adjuvant medication that may be used in conjunction with an analgesic to manage a patient's pain is:

25. The usual dosage of on-demand morphine in the PCA is:

26. Complete the following about analgesics.
    a. A priority nursing intervention specifically for the patient with an epidural analgesic infusion is:
    b. A priority nursing assessment for all patients before and while receiving analgesics is:
    c. To prevent accidental infusion of a drug intended for IV use, not epidural injection, you should:
    d. What medications are commonly used for epidural analgesia?

Copyright © 2019, Elsevier Inc. All Rights Reserved.

27. Identify an intervention that a nurse should implement to adapt or alter the environment to promote a patient's comfort.

28. A patient who may experience phantom pain is someone who has:

29. The term for patient-controlled oral analgesia is:

_____.

30. Whenever possible, the best way to evaluate the effectiveness of pain management is to:

_____.

31. The ABCDE approach to pain assessment and management is:
    A
    B
    C
    D
    E

32. Concomitant symptoms associated with pain include:

33. Identify whether the following statements are true or false.
    a. Nurses can allow their own misconceptions about or interpretations of the pain experience to affect their willingness to intervene for their patient.

    True _____ False _____

    b. The degree and quality of pain are related to the patient's definition of pain.

    True _____ False _____

    c. When patients are experiencing pain, they will not hesitate to inform you.

    True _____ False _____

    d. Fatigue decreases a patient's perception of pain.

    True _____ False _____

    e. A nurse should provide descriptive words for a patient to assist in assessing the quality of the pain.

    True _____ False _____

    f. Pain assessment can be delegated to assistive personnel.

    True _____ False _____

    g. Large doses of opioids for the terminally ill patient will hasten the onset of death.

    True _____ False _____

    h. Health care providers will initially order higher doses than needed for patients with cancer pain.

    True _____ False _____

    i. The Joint Commission (TJC) has a standard that requires health care workers to assess all patients for pain.

    True _____ False _____

    j. Pain is a normal part of aging.

    True _____ False _____

    k. Nurses should anticipate that higher doses of oral opioids will be ordered after patients are converted from the IV form.

    True _____ False _____

    l. The least invasive pain management therapy should be tried first.

    True _____ False _____

Copyright © 2019, Elsevier Inc. All Rights Reserved.

34. Which of the following usually result in better coping with the pain experience? Select all that apply.
   a. Presence of loved one/family members or friends

   _____

   b. Restful sleep _____

   c. Prior bad experience with pain _____

   d. High anxiety levels _____

   e. Depression _____

   f. Internal loci of control _____

35. Indicate three factors that contribute to older adults having their pain inadequately assessed and managed.

36. Identify which aspect of a patient's pain is being assessed with the following questions.

   a. How long has the pain lasted? _____

   b. Where do you feel the pain? _____

   c. What activity caused the pain? _____

   d. Is there something that lessens the pain? _____

37. For the QSEN competency of Teamwork and Collaboration, who are the other members of the health care team who may be involved in the patient's pain relief plan?

38. The patient is going to receive a local anesthetic prior to wound suturing. Which medications do you anticipate could be used?

39. The patient has a PCA pump in place and is sedated and not easily aroused. What should you do?

40. Which of the following are true regarding the use of analgesic patches for a patient with cancer pain? Select all that apply.
   a. The drug often takes 12–24 hours to take effect.

   _____

   b. Immediate-release opioids are not needed initially. _____

   c. Patients should avoid hot showers. _____

   d. Fentanyl is often used in the patches. _____

   e. A continuous-drip morphine is used at the same time. _____

Select the best answer for each of the following questions:

41. A patient is experiencing pain that is not being managed by analgesics given by the oral or intramuscular routes. Epidural analgesia is initiated. The nurse is alert for a complication of this treatment and observes the patient for:
   1. diarrhea.
   2. hypertension.
   3. urinary retention.
   4. an increased respiratory rate.

42. A patient had a laparoscopic procedure this morning and is requesting a pain medication. The nurse assesses the patient's vital signs and decides to withhold the medication based on the finding of:
   1. Temperature = 99°F, rectally.
   2. Pulse rate = 90 beats per minute, regular.
   3. Respirations = 9 per minute, shallow.
   4. Blood pressure = 130/80 mm Hg, consistent with prior reading.

43. A nurse is working with an older adult population in the extended care facility. Many of the patients experience discomfort associated with arthritis and have analgesics prescribed. In administering an analgesic medication to an older adult patient, the nurse should:
   1. give the medication when the pain increases in severity.
   2. combine opioids for a greater effect.
   3. use the IM route whenever possible.
   4. give the medication before activities or procedures.

44. One of the patients that a nurse is working with on an outpatient basis at the local clinic has mild osteoarthritis. The patient has no known allergies to any medications, so the nurse anticipates that the physician will prescribe:
   1. amitriptyline.
   2. butorphanol.
   3. ibuprofen.
   4. morphine.

45. An adolescent has been carried to the sidelines of the soccer field after experiencing a twisted ankle. The level of acute pain is identified as low to moderate. The nurse observes that the patient has:
   1. pupil constriction.
   2. diaphoresis.
   3. a decreased heart rate.
   4. a decreased respiratory rate.

Copyright © 2019, Elsevier Inc. All Rights Reserved.

46. A nurse on the pediatric unit is finding that it is sometimes difficult to determine the presence and severity of pain in very young patients. The nurse recognizes that toddlers may be experiencing pain when they have:
1. an increased appetite.
2. a relaxed posture.
3. an increased degree of cooperation.
4. disturbances in their sleep patterns.

47. A patient on the oncology unit is experiencing severe pain associated with his cancer. Although analgesics have been prescribed and administered, the patient is having "breakthrough pain." The nurse anticipates that his treatment will include:
1. the use of a placebo.
2. experimental medications.
3. an increase in the opioid dose.
4. administration of medications every hour.

48. A patient is experiencing pain that is being treated with a fentanyl transdermal patch. The nurse advises this patient to:
1. avoid exposure to the sun.
2. change the patch site every 2 hours.
3. apply a heating pad over the site.
4. expect immediate pain relief when the patch is applied.

49. A patient is experiencing severe pain and has been placed on a morphine drip. During the patient's assessment, the nurse finds that the patient's respiratory rate is 6 breaths per minute and shallow. The nurse anticipates that the patient will receive:
1. naloxone.
2. morphine.
3. incentive spirometry.
4. no additional treatment for this expected response.

50. The patient is in the dental office to have a tooth extraction. During the procedure, the dentist provides the patient with headphones to listen to music. This is an example of:
1. imagery.
2. biofeedback.
3. distraction.
4. cutaneous stimulation.

51. A nurse is working for an oncology unit in the medical center. All of the patients experience pain that requires management. The nurse should visit first with the patient who is also exhibiting signs of:
1. anxiety.
2. fatigue.
3. distraction.
4. depression.

52. For a patient with a consistent level of discomfort, the most effective pain relief is achieved with administration of analgesics:
1. PRN.
2. every 3–4 hours.
3. every 12 hours.
4. around the clock.

53. Which of the following orders would the nurse question for the patient who has an epidural infusion for pain relief?
1. Use of pulse oximetry
2. Tubing changes every 24 hours
3. An order for a sedative
4. Use of fentanyl in the infusion

54. Because of the possible cardiovascular and neurological effects, which of the following analgesic orders for an older adult patient with mild arthritis pain should be questioned?
1. Acetaminophen
2. Aspirin
3. Ibuprofen
4. Hydromorphone

STUDY GROUP QUESTIONS

• How can a nurse use a holistic approach to assist a patient in achieving comfort?
• What is pain?
• What are the physiological components of the pain experience?
• How may a patient respond, physiologically and behaviorally, to a pain experience?
• What factors influence the pain experience?
• How are acute and chronic pain different?
• How should a nurse assess a patient's pain?
• How may a patient characterize pain?
• What nonpharmacological measures may be used to relieve pain?
• What interventions may a nurse implement to promote comfort and relieve pain?
• What pharmacological measures are available for pain relief?
• What actions should a nurse take if comfort or pain relief measures are not effective?
• What information should be included in patient/family teaching for pain control or relief?

STUDY CHART

Create a study chart to describe the *Factors Influencing Pain and Comfort* that identifies how age, gender, neurological function, culture, spirituality, meaning of pain, and previous experience of a patient alter the pain experience.

Create a study chart that includes the dosages, routes, and nursing implications for common nonopioids and opioids.

Copyright © 2019, Elsevier Inc. All Rights Reserved.

35 Nutrition

PRELIMINARY READING

Chapter 35, pp. 972–1017

CASE STUDIES

1. You are working with a patient who is being discharged from the acute care unit after a heart attack (myocardial infarction). The patient's primary care provider has prescribed medical nutrition therapy, with a diet that is low in sodium and saturated fat. The patient comes from a family where food plays an important role in traditional culture practices.
   a. What do you need to know about the patient and the family to assist in dietary planning?
   b. How can you assist this patient to meet the prescribed dietary requirements?

2. A pregnant woman is at the medical office for a prenatal checkup. What nutritional recommendations should be provided to this patient?

3. You are working in a home care agency and have a large older adult patient population. In planning care, what nutritional considerations should be taken into account for these patients?

4. As an occupational health nurse, you are concerned with positive health behaviors for the employees. You have noticed that some of the workers are overweight.
   a. Identify the nursing diagnosis and general goals based upon your observation.
   b. What should you include in a teaching plan to promote nutritional health for the employees?

CHAPTER REVIEW

Match the description/definition in Column A with the correct term in Column B.

	Column A	Column B
_____	1. Increase in blood glucose level	a. Anabolism
_____	2. Breakdown of food products into smaller particles	b. Hypoglycemia
_____	3. Building of more complex substances from smaller particles	c. Digestion
_____	4. All biochemical and physiological processes	d. Anthropometry
_____	5. Organic substances present in small amounts in food that are essential for life	e. Catabolism
_____	6. Inorganic elements that act as catalysts in biochemical reactions	f. Nutrients
_____	7. Chemical substances that provide nourishment and affect metabolic and nutritive processes	g. Minerals
_____	8. Breakdown of complex body substances into simpler substances	h. Metabolism
_____	9. Decrease in blood glucose level	i. Hyperglycemia
_____	10. Measurement of size and makeup of body at specific sites	j. Vitamins

Copyright © 2019, Elsevier Inc. All Rights Reserved.

Complete the following:

11. Identify an example of a nutrition objective from *Healthy People 2020*.

12. For vitamins:
    a. Which vitamin is synthesized by the body?
    b. What are the fat-soluble vitamins?
    c. Identify an example of an antioxidant vitamin.

13. Identify whether the following represent carbohydrates, proteins, or fats.

    a. Starches _____

    b. Meats _____

    c. Linoleic acid _____

    d. Fiber _____

    e. 9 kcal/g of energy _____

    f. Amino acids _____

    g. Fruits _____

14. For patients with alterations in bowel elimination, identify which type of fiber should be recommended:

    a. Prevention of diarrhea: _____

    b. Prevention of constipation: _____

15. What information can you provide to an individual at a health fair who is interested in general nutritional guidelines?

16. Provide an example of an alternative dietary pattern.

17. a. Water makes up _____% of the total body weight.

    b. Describe the functions of water in the body.

18. What are the benefits of breastfeeding?

19. For each area of nutritional assessment, identify specific elements to pursue with the patient.
    a. Food and nutrient intake
    b. Physical examination
    c. Anthropometric measurements

20. Which of the following are indicators of malnutrition? Select all that apply.

    a. Listlessness _____

    b. Straight arms and legs _____

    c. Some fat under the skin _____

    d. Paresthesia _____

    e. Bow legs _____

    f. Rapid heart rate _____

    g. No palpable masses _____

    h. Apathy _____

    i. Dry, scaly skin _____

    j. Reddish-pink mucous membranes _____

    k. Spongy gums with marginal redness _____

    l. Surface papillae present on the tongue _____

    m. Pale conjunctivae _____

    n. Corneal xerosis _____

    o. Firm, pink nails _____

    p. Calf tenderness and tingling _____

21. A nurse calculates a patient's body mass index (BMI) by dividing the weight in kilograms by the height in square meters. If the patient weighs 180 pounds and is 6 feet tall, what is the BMI?

22. A neurogenic cause of dysphagia is:

    _____

    A myogenic cause is: _____

23. Common signs or symptoms of food-borne illnesses are:

24. A nurse on an acute care unit is concerned about the patient's appetite.
    a. What are the stressors in the environment that have an impact upon a patient's nutritional intake?
    b. Identify at least two interventions that should be implemented by the nurse to promote the patient's appetite.

Copyright © 2019, Elsevier Inc. All Rights Reserved.

25. Identify the interventions that a nurse should implement for the patient who is experiencing dysphagia.

26. An advantage of enteral nutrition over parenteral nutrition is that enteral nutrition:

27. Regarding enteral tube feedings:
    a. What are the contraindications to nasogastric tube placement?
    b. The most serious complication of tube feedings is:

    c. To avoid this complication, the nurse should:

    d. Displacement of a jejunostomy tube can lead to:

    e. The nasogastric tube becomes clogged. The nurse should:
    f. Intermittent nasogastric feeding tubes are clamped/closed to prevent:
    g. The method of choice for long-term enteral feeding for the patient who has not had upper GI surgery is:

28. On the food label pictured, what is/are the possible concerns?

Nutrition Facts

Serving Size: 1/2 cup (114 g)
Servings Per Container: 4

Amount per Serving

Calories 260
Calories from Fat 120

	% Daily Value*
Total Fat 13 g	20%
Saturated Fat 5 g	25%
Trans Fat 0 g	
Cholesterol 30 mg	10%
Sodium 660 mg	28%
Total Carbohydrate 31 g	11%
Dietary Fiber 0 g	0%
Sugars 5 g	
Protein 5 g	

Vitamin A 4%	•	Vitamin C 1%
Calcium 15%	•	Iron 4%

*Percents (%) of a Daily Value are based on a 2,000 calorie diet. Your Daily Values may vary higher or lower depending on your calorie needs.

Nutrient	2,000 calories	2,500 calories
Total Fat	<65 g	<80 g
Saturated Fat	<20 g	<25 g
Cholesterol	<300 mg	<300 mg
Sodium	<2,400 mg	<2,400 mg
Total Carbohydrate	300 g	375 g
Dietary Fiber	25 g	30 g

1 g Fat = 9 calories
1 g Carbohydrate = 4 calories
1 g Protein = 4 calories

29. Identify foods that are choking hazards for toddlers.

30. What are the contributing factors to adolescent obesity and nutritional deficiencies?

31. The appearance of the gastric aspirate for a patient who has been fasting is:

32. A parenteral nutrition formula that is hyperosmolar (greater than 10% dextrose) should be administered through a _____ venous line.

33. A patient will be receiving parenteral nutrition (PN). Identify the following:
    a. The main reason for use of PN:
    b. A major nursing goal for the patient receiving PN:
    c. A nursing intervention to assist the patient in the prevention of metabolic complications related to PN therapy:
    d. Guidelines and precautions for lipid infusions:

34. Identify a dietary measure that should be implemented for a patient without teeth or with ill-fitting dentures.

35. A screening tool for older adults is the Mini Nutritional Assessment (MNA). Select all of the following correct statements about this tool.

    a. It is an 18-item tool. _____

    b. There are 4 sections to complete. _____

    c. The sections are divided into screening and assessment items. _____

    d. A score above 12 indicates a positive nutritional assessment. _____

    e. Anthropometric measures are required for the screening. _____

36. Indicate whether the following statements are true or false.
    a. Infants require more protein than adults.

       True _____ False _____

    b. 17.5% of children ages 6–11 years are classified as obese in the United States.

       True _____ False _____

Copyright © 2019, Elsevier Inc. All Rights Reserved.

37. What is the purpose of the ChooseMyPlate program?

38. What interventions should be implemented for a patient who is receiving enteral feedings? Select all that apply.
   a. Keep the head of the bed elevated to 30–45 degrees. _____
   b. Withhold the feeding if the residual is 50–100 mL. _____
   c. Tube placement is confirmed before feedings by monitoring the pH of aspirate. _____
   d. Gastric residual volume is measured daily. _____
   e. Continuous feedings are administered through an infusion pump. _____
   f. Tubing should be flushed with 200 mL of water before and after each feeding. _____

39. What are the benefits of the DASH diet?

40. Complete a brief narrative documentation example that includes the following:
   10 Fr nasogastric tube, left side insertion, verification of placement, patient tolerance of procedure

41. The nurse is going to provide a continuous enteral feeding. Place the following steps in the correct order. Note: Certain steps have been completed, such as hand hygiene.
   a. Label the time the bag was hung. _____
   b. Verify the order. _____
   c. Pour the feeding into the bag. _____
   d. Bring the formula to room temperature. _____
   e. Check the expiration date on the formula. _____
   f. Remove cap on tubing and connect distal end of administration set tubing to feeding tube. _____
   g. Thread tubing through feeding pump; set rate on pump and turn on. _____

42. a. Patients with dysphagia will always cough when food enters the airway.
      True _____ False _____
   b. Verification of enteral tube placement can be delegated to nursing assistive personnel.
      True _____ False _____
   c. Preparation for enteral feeding includes clean technique.
      True _____ False _____
   d. The nasogastric tube should be iced before insertion.
      True _____ False _____

43. Complete the following:

Foodborne Disease	Organism	Food Source	Symptoms
E. coli			
Hepatitis			
Salmonellosis			

44. The standard for weighing patients is to:

45. Put the steps for aspiration prevention in the correct order.
   a. Provide verbal coaching: remind patient to chew and think about swallowing. _____
   b. Ask patient to remain sitting upright for at least 30–60 minutes. _____
   c. Place the patient in a chair or raise the head of the bed to an upright, seated position. _____
   d. Have patient assume chin-tuck position. Remind patient to not tilt head backward when eating or while drinking. _____
   e. Using penlight and tongue blade, gently inspect mouth for pockets of food. _____
   f. Add thickener to thin liquids to create desired consistency per SLP assessment. _____

46. What documentation should be done after NG tube insertion?

Copyright © 2019, Elsevier Inc. All Rights Reserved.

47. How should an enteral tube be removed?

Select the best answer for each of the following questions:

48. A nurse is working with a patient who requires an increase in protein in the diet, but the patient does not like meat. The nurse recommends:
    1. fruit.
    2. cereals.
    3. beans.
    4. vegetables.

49. A nurse is talking with a community resident who has gone to the health fair. The resident tells the nurse that he takes a lot of extra vitamins every day. Because of the greater potential for toxicity, the resident is advised not to exceed the dietary guidelines for:
    1. vitamin A.
    2. vitamin B_1.
    3. vitamin B_{12}.
    4. folic acid.

50. A nurse is working with a patient who is a lactovegetarian. The food that is selected as appropriate for this dietary pattern is:
    1. fish.
    2. milk.
    3. eggs.
    4. poultry.

51. A patient states that he does not eat fish anymore. An appropriate follow-up question by the nurse is which of the following?
    1. "Why don't you like fish?"
    2. "What do you believe caused you to lose interest in fish?"
    3. "Fish makes you feel ill in some way?"
    4. "Aren't you aware that fish is a valuable source of nutrients?"

52. A nurse is preparing to insert a nasogastric tube for enteral feedings. The nurse recognizes that this intervention is used when the patient:
    1. has a gag reflex.
    2. is not able to metabolize nutrients.
    3. is slow to eliminate food.
    4. is not able to swallow foods.

53. A nurse is preparing the enteral feeding for a patient who has a nasogastric tube in place. The most effective method that the nurse can use to check for placement of a nasogastric tube is to:
    1. perform a pH analysis of aspirated gastric secretions.
    2. measure the visible tubing exiting from the nose.
    3. inject air into the tube and auscultate over the stomach.
    4. place the end of the tube into water and observe for bubbling.

54. Prior to insertion of an NG tube, the nurse assesses that the patient has abdominal pain and distention. This indicates that:
    1. the tube should be inserted quickly.
    2. feedings are contraindicated at this time.
    3. a gastrostomy tube should be inserted.
    4. there is a risk for tracheobronchial tree insertion.

55. A patient tells the nurse that she is a vegan. Which of the following vitamin supplements is needed to promote health for this patient?
    1. Niacin
    2. Vitamin C
    3. Thiamine
    4. Vitamin B_{12}

56. A nurse is assigned to make home visits to a number of patients. Of the patients that the nurse visits, the patient with the greatest risk of a nutritional deficiency is the patient with:
    1. decreased metabolic requirements.
    2. an alteration in dietary schedule and intake.
    3. a body weight that is 1% over the ideal weight.
    4. a weight loss of 2% within the past 6 months.

57. After surgery, a patient is having her dietary intake advanced. After a period of NPO, the patient is placed on a clear liquid diet. What food does the nurse request for the patient?
    1. Milk
    2. Soup
    3. Custard
    4. Popsicles

58. Which of the following types of fluid are the most difficult to swallow for a patient with dysphagia?
    1. Thin liquids
    2. Nectar-like liquids
    3. Honey-like liquids
    4. Spoon-thick liquids

59. A patient on the unit has an enteral tube in place for feedings. When the nurse enters the room, the patient says that he is experiencing cramps and nausea. The nurse should:
    1. cool the formula.
    2. remove the tube.
    3. use a more concentrated formula.
    4. decrease the administration rate temporarily.

Copyright © 2019, Elsevier Inc. All Rights Reserved.

60. Which of the following statements made by the parent of an infant indicates the need for additional teaching?
    1. "I'll wait to give the baby regular cow's milk until he is a year old."
    2. "I'll start with cereal as the first solid food that I give to the baby after about 6 months."
    3. "I'll add a little honey to the baby's bottle to help him digest the formula."
    4. "I'll wait a few days in between giving the baby any new foods."

61. For the family that cans food at home, there is a need for specific instruction about ways to prevent
    1. botulism.
    2. *E. coli.*
    3. salmonellosis.
    4. listeriosis.

62. The individual with the highest percentage of water in the body is a(n):
    1. infant.
    2. obese patient.
    3. adolescent.
    4. older adult.

63. A patient with a gastrostomy has a gastric residual volume (GRV) of 100 mL. Unless contraindicated by agency policy, the nurse should:
    1. request an order for a chest x-ray.
    2. alter the type of feeding being given.
    3. request an order for an antidiarrheal agent.
    4. return the aspirated contents to the stomach.

64. A nurse is monitoring a patient's laboratory reports. Which of the following, if decreased, is indicative of anemia?
    1. BUN
    2. Creatinine
    3. Albumin
    4. Hemoglobin

65. A nurse is instructing the family of a patient who is on a high fiber diet to include more:
    1. mashed potatoes.
    2. well-cooked noodles.
    3. fresh fruits.
    4. cheese.

66. A nurse recognizes that a patient on a low cholesterol diet requires additional teaching if he indicates that he eats which of the following?
    1. Oatmeal
    2. Pastries
    3. Dried fruits
    4. Green peppers

67. For a patient who is receiving medications via the feeding tube, which of the following actions is appropriate?
    1. Flush the tube with water before and after each medication is administered.
    2. Mix the medications with the formula.
    3. Administer all of the medications together.
    4. Obtain orders for the injectable form of each medication.

68. To prevent the presence of *E. coli* in food, a nurse specifically instructs a patient and family to:
    1. carefully can foods at home.
    2. boil shellfish completely.
    3. cook ground beef well.
    4. keep dairy products refrigerated.

69. A nurse is visiting a patient in the home and notes that additional teaching is required if the patient is observed:
    1. cooking poultry to 180°F.
    2. thawing frozen foods at room temperature.
    3. discarding all foods that may be spoiled.
    4. cleaning the inside of the refrigerator regularly.

70. Continuous feedings are ordered for a patient with a nasogastric tube. Unless the agency specifies otherwise, the nurse should:
    1. dilute the feedings with water.
    2. infuse the feedings over the course of 1–2 hours.
    3. measure gastric residual volume every 4–6 hours.
    4. increase feedings by 100–150 mL per feeding every 8 hours.

71. Which one of the following foods is avoided by the patient on a gluten-free diet?
    1. Cow's milk
    2. Wheat cereal
    3. Canned fruit
    4. Coffee

72. During the insertion of a nasogastric tube, the unit nurse manager is observing the new nurse graduate. Correction is required when the new nurse:
    1. has the patient flex the head after the tube passes the nasopharynx.
    2. rotates the tube 180 degrees during the insertion.
    3. encourages the patient to swallow as the tube moves along.
    4. advances the tube during patient inspiration.

Copyright © 2019, Elsevier Inc. All Rights Reserved.

STUDY GROUP QUESTIONS

- What are the basic principles of nutrition?
- What body processes are involved in the intake, use, and elimination of foods?
- What are the six major nutrients and their purposes?
- What are the current recommendations for daily nutritional intake?
- How do nutritional needs change across the life span?
- How does culture/ethnicity influence dietary intake?
- What are some common alternative food patterns?
- How should a nurse assess a patient's nutritional status?
- What patients are at a greater risk for nutritional deficiencies?
- What nursing diagnoses may be appropriate for patients with nutritional alterations?
- How does a nurse assist patients to meet nutritional needs in the health promotion, acute care, and restorative care settings?

- What special diets may be prescribed for individuals?
- What are the nursing procedures for implementation of enteral and parenteral nutrition?
- What guidelines and precautions should be considered by a nurse in assisting a patient with enteral or parenteral nutrition?
- What general information should be included for patients/families for promotion or restoration of an adequate nutritional intake?
- How can the nurse assess for and assist a patient with dysphagia?
- What measures can be taken to prevent aspiration?

STUDY CHART

Create a study chart to describe the *Six Nutrients* that identifies the uses of each in the body and examples of food sources: carbohydrates, proteins, lipids, vitamins, minerals, and water.

Copyright © 2019, Elsevier Inc. All Rights Reserved.

36 Urinary Elimination

Chapter 36, pp. 1018–1058

CASE STUDIES

1. A patient is going to the medical center for an intravenous pyelogram (IVP).
   a. What nursing assessments and patient teaching should be completed before this test is performed?
   b. What are the nurse's responsibilities for the patient following an IVP?

2. You will be working with unlicensed assistive personnel in an extended care setting.
   a. What urinary care may be safely delegated by a nurse?

3. On an acute care unit, a patient is to have her catheter removed. The primary nurse tells you that all that is necessary is to "cut it, wait for the balloon to deflate, and pull it out."
   a. How will you proceed with this catheter removal?

4. A clean-voided or midstream urine specimen is required from a male patient. He is able to perform activities of daily living, including hygienic care.
   a. How will you teach this patient to obtain the specimen?

5. A patient had surgery and an incontinent urinary diversion was created.
   a. What are the special needs of this patient and the interventions that you will implement?

6. The patient tells you that she is not sure whether she may have a urinary tract infection.
   a. What information can you provide to her about UTIs?
   b. What can she do to prevent UTIs?

CHAPTER REVIEW

Match the description/definition in Column A with the correct term in Column B.

	Column A	*Column B*
_____	1. Accumulation of urine in the bladder because of inability to empty bladder completely	a. Urgency
_____	2. Painful or difficult urination	b. Hematuria
_____	3. Difficulty in initiating urination	c. Oliguria
_____	4. Volume of urine remaining in the bladder after voiding	d. Retention
_____	5. Feeling the need to void immediately	e. Nocturia
_____	6. Voiding large amounts of urine	f. Frequency
_____	7. Urination, particularly excessive, at night	g. Dysuria
_____	8. Presence of blood in the urine	h. Residual urine
_____	9. Voiding very often	i. Hesitancy
_____	10. Diminished urinary output in relation to fluid intake	j. Polyuria

159

Copyright © 2019, Elsevier Inc. All Rights Reserved.

Complete the following:

11. An example of a noninvasive procedure that may be used to examine the urinary system is:

12. What are the indications for the use of intermittent and indwelling urinary catheterization?

13. What positions may be used for catheterization of a female patient?

14. a. The recommended daily fluid intake for dilution of urine, promotion of micturition, and flushing the urethra of microorganisms is:

    b. The minimum urinary output for an adult is
    _____ per hour.

15. Provide an example of how each of the following factors may influence urination.
    a. Sociocultural
    b. Fluid intake
    c. Medications

16. Identify how the following pathological conditions can influence urination:
    a. Arthritis
    b. Diabetes mellitus
    c. Prostate enlargement

17. a. The type of urinary incontinence that results from increased intra-abdominal pressure with leakage of a small amount of urine is called:

    b. The treatment for this type of incontinence includes:

18. Which of the following are the expected characteristics of a normal urine specimen? Select all that apply.

    a. pH 10 _____

    b. Protein 4 mg/100 mL _____

    c. Presence of glucose _____

    d. Specific gravity 1.2 _____

    e. Amber color _____

    f. Thick, cloudy _____

    g. Ketones _____

19. What is a priority when managing a patient's condom catheter?

20. To maintain a patient's dignity and self-esteem when assisting with urinary elimination, the nurse makes sure to:

21. The catheter is accidentally inserted into the patient's vagina. What should you do?

22. Which of the following statements are correct for urinary diversions? Select all that apply.

    a. A ureterostomy is a continent diversion. _____

    b. Continent diversions have internal pouches created to store urine. _____

    c. Patients with urinary diversions cannot maintain normal activity. _____

23. For an ambulatory patient on strict intake and output, identify how urinary output can be measured.

24. Identify a method that a nurse may implement to stimulate a patient to void:

25. To assist a patient to start and stop the urine stream, a nurse instructs the patient that a way to strengthen the pelvic floor muscles is by performing:

26. Identify the distance of catheter insertion:
    a. Female adult patient:
    b. Male adult patient:

27. Which of the following are appropriate techniques for indwelling catheter care? Select all that apply.
    a. Keep the drainage bag below the level of the bladder. _____

    b. Provide perineal care every two or three days. _____

    c. Cleanse in a direction toward the urinary meatus. _____

    d. Attach the drainage bag to the side rail of the bed. _____

    e. Open the connection at the drainage bag to obtain a urine specimen. _____

    f. Avoid having any kinks or dependent loops of tubing. _____

Copyright © 2019, Elsevier Inc. All Rights Reserved.

g. Drain urine from the bag before patient ambulation or exercise. _____

h. For the immobile patient, empty the drainage bag every 24 hours. _____

28. To prevent nocturia, a nurse instructs a patient to:

29. Identify how the mobility status of an older adult may influence urination.

30. Which of the following are expected signs or symptoms for a patient with acute onset urinary retention? Select all that apply.

   a. Tenderness over the symphysis pubis _____

   b. Hematuria _____

   c. Diaphoresis _____

   d. Oliguria _____

   e. Dysuria _____

   f. Incontinence _____

31. How can urinary infection (CAUTI) be prevented or reduced for a patient with an indwelling catheter?

32. Which of the following statements are correct regarding a cystoscopy? Select all that apply.

   a. The procedure may be performed under general anesthesia. _____

   b. Fluids are restricted before and during the procedure. _____

   c. Antibiotics are often ordered before and after the procedure. _____

   d. An informed consent is not required. _____

   e. The patient should lie still during the procedure. _____

   f. The patient is NPO if the test is performed with local anesthesia. _____

   g. Bed rest is usually indicated immediately after the test. _____

   h. Pink-tinged urine may be observed after the test. _____

   i. Fluid intake is encouraged after the test is completed. _____

33. During a physical assessment, what techniques are used to:
   a. Determine the presence of a kidney infection?
   b. Assess the bladder?

34. Identify the following for a bladder scanner:
   a. Use:
   b. When to measure:

35. Identify the characteristic of the urine for a patient with:
   a. Daily administration of furosemide (Lasix):

   _____

   b. Liver disease: _____

   c. Urinary tract infection: _____

36. Urinary specimens for analysis should be sent to the laboratory within _____ hours of collection.

37. Place the following steps for a clean-catch specimen in the correct order:

   a. Void in the toilet _____

   b. Provide instruction to the patient _____

   c. Void in a sterile urine cup _____

   d. Cleanse the urinary meatus _____

   e. Stop the urine stream _____

38. The patient is going to have a computerized axial tomography (CT) scan to identify the possible presence of calculi. Identify the following:
   a. Preparation before the test:
   b. Care following the test:

Copyright © 2019, Elsevier Inc. All Rights Reserved.

39. a. Current evidence shows silver-coated catheters may reduce the incidence of CAUTI for short-term use.

    True _____ False _____

    b. Make every attempt to remove catheters as soon as a patient can void.

    True _____ False _____

    c. Empty the urine drainage bag when it is full.

    True _____ False _____

    d. The goal for intermittent catheterization is drainage of 400 mL of urine every 2–3 hours while awake.

    True _____ False _____

    e. The general guideline is to use the largest urinary catheter possible.

    True _____ False _____

    f. An indwelling catheter can be removed by cutting the tubing to deflate the balloon.

    True _____ False _____

    g. Self-catheterization by the patient at home is done with sterile technique.

    True _____ False _____

    h. Timed voiding is based upon a fixed schedule and not on the patient's urge to void.

    True _____ False _____

40. Identify the correct urinary catheter (single, double, or triple-lumen) to use for each of the following interventions:
    a. Indwelling catheter with bladder irrigation:
    b. Intermittent catheterization:
    c. Indwelling catheter:

41. What are the responsibilities of the nurse following the removal of a urinary catheter?

42. Identify the following for a suprapubic catheter:
    a. Purpose of insertion:
    b. Size of the catheter:
    c. Nursing care:

43. The patient has an incontinent urinary diversion and requires care of the stoma. Place the nursing actions in the correct order:
    a. Apply the pouch and press firmly into place. _____

    b. Cleanse the skin around the stoma. _____

    c. Remove the protective backing from the adhesive surface on the pouch _____

    d. Measure the stoma. _____

    e. Cut an opening in the pouch. _____

44. What type of medications are used to treat urgency urinary incontinence?

45. What needs to be recorded after the insertion of an indwelling urinary catheter?

46. Put the steps of measurement with a bladder scanner in the correct order.
    a. Apply light pressure, keep scanner head steady, and point it slightly downward toward bladder. Press and release the scan button. _____

    b. Palpate patient's symphysis pubis. Apply generous amount of ultrasound gel (or, if available, a bladder scan gel pad) to midline abdomen 2.5–4 cm (1–1.5 inches) above symphysis pubis. _____

    c. Turn on scanner per manufacturer guidelines. _____

    d. Help patient to supine position with head slightly elevated. Raise bed to appropriate working height. If side rails are raised, lower side rail on working side. _____

    e. Set gender designation per manufacturer guidelines. Designate women who have had a hysterectomy as male. _____

    f. Expose patient's lower abdomen. _____

    g. Place scanner head on gel, ensuring that scanner head is oriented per manufacturer guidelines. _____

    h. Wipe scanner head with alcohol pad or other cleaner and allow to air dry. _____

47. Hematuria is usually the result of:

48. The nurse is teaching the patient how to prevent UTIs. Identify all of the information that should be included in the instruction. Select all that apply.

    a. Cleanse the perineum from back to front. _____

    b. Void before and after sexual intercourse. _____

    c. Wear nylon underwear. _____

    d. Avoid bubble baths. _____

    e. Drink coffee or tea regularly. _____

    f. Try to empty the bladder completely with each voiding. _____

Copyright © 2019, Elsevier Inc. All Rights Reserved.

49. The patient is unable to void after catheter removal, has a sensation of not emptying, strains to void, or experiences small voiding amounts with increasing frequency. You should:

50. What are three possible questions to ask the patient to determine if there are any urinary symptoms present?

51. In the photo, what intervention is needed to have appropriate urinary drainage?

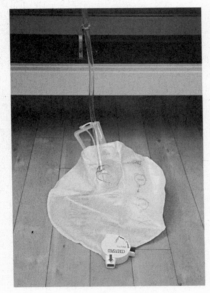

52. What lumen is used to inflate the catheter balloon?

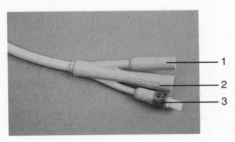

Select the best answer for each of the following questions:

53. The nurse recognizes that the initial intervention for a patient in any care setting who is found to be incontinent is:
    1. use of a mobility aid.
    2. intermittent catheterization.
    3. arranging a toilet schedule.
    4. administration of antimuscarinic medications.

54. The nurse is going to be catheterizing an average-size 9-year-old boy. The appropriate catheter size for this child is
    1. 5–6 Fr.
    2. 8–10 Fr.
    3. 12–14 Fr.
    4. 15–17 Fr.

55. For a patient with functional urinary incontinence, the difficulty is related to the patient's:
    1. inability to completely empty the bladder.
    2. lack of sensation of a full bladder.
    3. pressure during coughing or sneezing.
    4. difficulty in getting out of the chair and going to the toilet.

56. For the patient who has had a continent urinary reservoir created, the nurse instructs the patient that there will be a need to:
    1. catheterize the pouch 4–6 times/day.
    2. eliminate urine through the intestine.
    3. use the Valsalva maneuver to empty the pouch through the urethra.
    4. restrict the intake of fluids.

57. The nurse is going to explain to the new parents about toilet training. The parents are informed that control of voluntary voiding usually does not occur until the age of:
    1. 6–8 months old.
    2. 12–14 months old.
    3. 2–3 years old.
    4. 4–5 years old.

58. A patient on the medical unit is scheduled to have a 24-hour urine collection to diagnose a urinary disorder. The nurse should:
    1. note the start time on the container.
    2. have the patient void while defecating.
    3. start with the first voiding sample from the patient.
    4. continue with the test if a specimen is flushed away.

59. One of a nurse's assigned patients is experiencing urgency urinary incontinence (UI). The nurse anticipates a medication that may be ordered for this difficulty is:
    1. propantheline.
    2. oxybutynin.
    3. bethanechol.
    4. phenylpropanolamine.

163

Copyright © 2019, Elsevier Inc. All Rights Reserved.

60. Several patients in a long-term care unit have indwelling urinary catheters in place. A nurse is delegating catheter care to the nursing assistant. The nurse includes instruction in:
   1. using lotion on the perineal area.
   2. disinfecting the first 2–3 inches of the catheter every 2 hours.
   3. ensuring that the drainage bag is secured to the side rail.
   4. cleansing about 4 inches along the length of the catheter, proximal to distal.

61. For a renal ultrasound, the patient is instructed to:
   1. not eat or drink for 8 hours before.
   2. have a full bladder.
   3. complete bowel cleansing.
   4. not do anything out of his/her routine, as there is no special preparation for this procedure.

62. Prevention of infection is an outcome that is identified for a patient with a urinary alteration and an indwelling catheter. The nurse assists the patient to attain this outcome by:
   1. emptying the drainage bag daily.
   2. draining all urine after the patient ambulates.
   3. performing perineal care q8h and PRN.
   4. opening the drainage system only at the connector points to obtain specimens.

63. The patient's urine is uniformly red in color. The nurse suspects that it may be the result of a food or medication that the patient has ingested. Which of the following may have caused the urinary coloration?
   1. Phenazopyridine
   2. Blackberries
   3. Furosemide
   4. Oranges

64. A patient being seen at a urologist's office suffers from urge incontinence. The nurse anticipates that treatment for this difficulty will include:
   1. bladder surgery.
   2. catheterization.
   3. antimuscarinic drug therapy.
   4. electrical stimulation.

65. A patient had a laparoscopic procedure in the morning and is having difficulty voiding later that day. Before initiating invasive measures, the nurse intervenes by:
   1. administering a cholinergic agent.
   2. applying firm pressure over the perineal area.
   3. increasing the patient's daily fluid intake to 3000 mL.
   4. rinsing the perineal area with warm water.

66. To determine the possibility of a renal problem, a patient is scheduled to have an intravenous pyelogram (IVP). Immediately after the procedure, a nurse will need to evaluate the patient's response and be alert to:
   1. an infection in the urinary bladder.
   2. an allergic reaction to the contrast material.
   3. urinary suppression from injury to kidney tissues.
   4. incontinence from paralysis of the urinary sphincter.

67. A unit manager is evaluating the care that has been given to a patient by a new nursing staff member. The manager determines that the staff member has implemented an appropriate technique for a clean-voided urine specimen collection if:
   1. fluids were restricted before the collection.
   2. sterile gloves were applied for the procedure.
   3. the specimen was collected after the initial stream of urine had passed.
   4. the specimen was placed in a clean container and then placed in the utility room.

68. A patient at the urology clinic is diagnosed with reflex incontinence. This problem was identified by the patient's statement of experiencing:
   1. a constant dribbling of urine.
   2. an urge to void and not enough time to reach the bathroom.
   3. an uncontrollable loss of urine when coughing or sneezing.
   4. no urge to void and being unaware of bladder fullness.

69. A female patient has an order for urinary catheterization. A nursing student will be evaluated by the instructor on the insertion technique. The student is identified as implementing appropriate technique if:
   1. the catheter is advanced 2–3 inches.
   2. the balloon is inflated before insertion.
   3. both hands are kept sterile throughout the procedure.
   4. the catheter is reinserted if it is accidentally placed in the vagina.

70. A patient is diagnosed with prostate enlargement. The nurse is alert to a specific indication of this problem when finding that the patient has:
   1. chills.
   2. cloudy urine.
   3. polyuria.
   4. bladder distention.

Copyright © 2019, Elsevier Inc. All Rights Reserved.

71. Stress urinary incontinence is associated with:
    1. irritation of the bladder.
    2. neurological trauma.
    3. alcohol or caffeine ingestion
    4. coughing or sneezing.

72. For patients with uncontrolled diabetes mellitus, a nurse anticipates that the patients will experience:
    1. dribbling.
    2. hesitancy.
    3. polyuria.
    4. hematuria.

73. A nurse recognizes that one of the specific purposes of intermittent catheterization is for:
    1. prevention of obstruction.
    2. assessment of residual urine.
    3. urinary drainage during surgical procedures.
    4. recording of output for comatose patients.

74. A nurse notes that there is no urine in a drainage bag since it was emptied 2 hours ago. The nurse should first:
    1. remove the catheter.
    2. provide additional fluids.
    3. check for kinks or bends in the tubing.
    4. apply external pressure on the patient's bladder.

75. The best way to remove urine from a patient's skin is for the nurse to use:
    1. alcohol.
    2. mild soap.
    3. an antibacterial agent.
    4. a hydrogen peroxide mix.

76. A nurse manager is observing a new nurse staff member provide care for a patient with a condom catheter. The manager determines that correction and additional instruction are required for the new employee if the staff nurse is observed:
    1. draping the patient and exposing only the genitalia for the application.
    2. securing the urinary drainage bag to the patient or lower bed frame.
    3. using barrier cream to the patient's penis.
    4. clipping excess hair at the base of the penis.

77. A patient who is taking phenazopyridine needs to be instructed that a specific side effect of this medication is that:
    1. the urine will turn orange.
    2. there will be an increased urinary frequency.
    3. back pain will be moderately severe.
    4. occasional dizziness may be experienced.

78. A nurse anticipates that a treatment option for a patient with functional incontinence will include:
    1. catheterization.
    2. bladder training.
    3. electrical stimulation.
    4. hormone replacement.

STUDY GROUP QUESTIONS

- What is the normal anatomy and physiology of the urinary system?
- What factors may influence urination?
- What are some common urinary elimination problems, their causes, and patient signs and symptoms?
- How do growth and development influence urinary function and patterns?
- How can urinary drainage be surgically altered, and why would an alteration be necessary?
- What measures may be implemented to prevent infection in the urinary tract?
- How does a nurse assess a patient's urinary function/elimination?
- What noninvasive and invasive procedures may be used to determine urinary function?
- What diagnostic tests are used to determine the characteristics of urine?
- What are the expected characteristics of urine?
- What nursing interventions are appropriate for promoting urination in the health care and home care settings?
- What information should be included in teaching patients/families about promotion of urination and prevention of infection?
- How can a patient's personal feelings and concerns be respected while promoting urinary elimination?

Copyright © 2019, Elsevier Inc. All Rights Reserved.

37 Bowel Elimination

PRELIMINARY READING

Chapter 37, pp. 1059–1099

CASE STUDIES

1. You have arranged with your instructor and the home care agency to visit a 76-year-old woman. In completing your initial assessment, the patient tells you that she has been having difficulty over the past 2 years in "moving her bowels." She takes you to the bathroom, where she shows you a collection of over-the-counter laxatives and enemas. The patient also tells you that, since the death of her husband, she does not do a lot of cooking, relying on sandwiches and prepared foods.
   a. Based on this information, identify a nursing diagnosis, patient goal(s)/outcomes, and nursing interventions related to bowel elimination.

2. A patient is scheduled to have a colonoscopy performed.
   a. What are the screening guidelines for this procedure with respect to age group and frequency?
   b. Identify the patient teaching that is provided before the procedure.

CHAPTER REVIEW

Match the description/definition in Column A with the correct term in Column B.

	Column A	Column B
_____	1. Propulsion of food through the gastrointestinal (GI) tract	a. Stoma
_____	2. Agent used to empty the bowel	b. Flatus
_____	3. An increase in the number of stools and the passage of liquid, unformed stools	c. Ileus
_____	4. Dilated rectal veins	d. Constipation
_____	5. Blood in the stool	e. Cathartic
_____	6. Artificial opening in the abdominal wall	f. Diarrhea
_____	7. Temporary cessation of peristalsis	g. Peristalsis
_____	8. Accumulated gas	h. Hemorrhoids
_____	9. Hard or dry stools, or decreased frequency	i. Melena
_____	10. Normal GI tract function, voluntary sphincter control	j. Defecation

Copyright © 2019, Elsevier Inc. All Rights Reserved.

Complete the following:

11. Constipation in the older adult is usually the result of:

12. What types of patients should be cautioned against straining during defecation and why?

13. a. A common cause of diarrhea in health care facilities is:
    b. This common occurrence can be prevented by:
    c. If persistent diarrhea occurs, a patient is at risk for:

14. The most frequently reported GI complaints are:

15. Provide an example of the effect that fecal incontinence can have on an individual.

16. Which of the following factors will interfere with bowel elimination and decrease peristalsis? Select all that apply.

    a. Slower esophageal emptying _____

    b. Eating raw vegetables _____

    c. Immobilization _____

    d. Consumption of lean meats _____

    e. Anxiety _____

    f. Emotional depression _____

    g. Abdominal surgery _____

    h. Use of antibiotics _____

    i. Food allergies _____

    j. Parkinson's disease _____

    k. Use of opiates _____

    l. Drinking fruit juices _____

    m. Tube feedings _____

17. Discuss how a patient's cultural background may influence care for elimination needs.

18. Identify a risk factor for colon cancer.

19. Identify two nursing interventions for a patient who is experiencing:
    a. Constipation
    b. Diarrhea

20. Provide an example of how each of the following factors influences bowel elimination.
    a. Positioning
    b. Pregnancy
    c. Diagnostic tests
    d. Diet
    e. Personal habits

21. How can a nurse promote comfort for a patient with hemorrhoids?

22. Identify at least three areas included in a GI assessment.

23. Enema administration:
    a. What is the correct position for an adult patient to receive an enema?
    b. The enema tube is inserted as follows:

       Adult: _____ inches or _____ cm

       Child: _____ inches or _____ cm
    c. The height of the bag for a regular adult enema

       should be _____ inches or _____ cm above the level of the anus.
    d. An enema that is used to treat patients with hyperkalemia is:
    e. A hypertonic enema works by:
    f. A commonly used over-the-counter hypertonic enema is:
    g. For a soapsuds enema, the only appropriate soap to use is:
    h. Provision of "enemas until clear" means:
    i. Following administration of an enema, what assessments should be made?
    j. The safest enema solution to use is:
    k. In a noncommercial enema, how much solution is used for:
       a. An adult
       b. A child who weighs 25 kg

24. The nurse anticipates that which of the osmotic laxatives could be prescribed for patients experiencing constipation: Select all that apply.

    a. Lactulose _____

    b. Loperamide _____

    c. Sorbitol _____

    d. Magnesium hydroxide _____

    e. Bisacodyl _____

    f. Polyethylene glycol _____

Copyright © 2019, Elsevier Inc. All Rights Reserved.

25. How is the QSEN competency for patient-centered care incorporated into the care of a patient with elimination needs?

26. A patient receiving tube feedings may experience diarrhea as a result of:

27. Identify what should be included in a focused assessment of a patient's bowel function.

28. For collection of fecal specimens:
   a. Identify how much is collected.
   b. What is done with the specimen after collection?

29. Which of the following are correct practices that should be included in the teaching plan for a patient with an ostomy? Select all that apply.
   a. Using creams around the peristomal skin _____
   b. Emptying the pouch when it is one-third to one-half full _____
   c. Washing the peristomal skin with a detergent soap _____
   d. Using sterile technique _____
   e. Anticipating a significant amount of bleeding _____
   f. Changing the entire pouching system daily _____
   g. Using the same manufacturer's flange and pouch _____
   h. Tracing stoma measurement on skin barrier and cut to size _____
   i. Applying a skin barrier around the stoma _____

30. Which of the following are expected findings? Select all that apply.
   a. Infant's yellow stool _____
   b. A defecation frequency greater than three times per day for an adult _____
   c. White-colored stool _____
   d. Tarry stool _____
   e. Soft, formed stool _____

31. When giving a patient a bedpan, the nurse should:

32. Select which of the following interventions may be delegated to assistive personnel.
   a. Digital removal of an impaction _____
   b. Non-medicated enema administration _____
   c. Pouching of a new ostomy _____
   d. Assisting the patient to use the bedpan _____

33. When determining placement of the nasogastric tube, it is expected that, if the tube is in the stomach, the gastric pH will be:

34. a. Clostridium difficile is transmitted by:
   b. Transmission of C. difficile can be prevented or reduced by:

35. Identify a positive outcome for a patient who has a colostomy.

36. Normal defecation in the acute- or long-term care environment may be promoted by:

37. Nasogastric tube irrigation is usually done with _____ mL of _____ (solution). Suction applied to the NG tube is usually _____.

38. Place the following steps for nasogastric tube insertion in the correct order:
   a. Have the patient drink water and swallow. _____
   b. Perform hand hygiene. _____
   c. Auscultate for bowel sounds. _____
   d. Insert the tube past the nasopharynx. _____
   e. Collect the equipment. _____
   f. Measure the distance to insert the tube. _____
   g. Ask the patient to talk. _____
   h. Identify the patient. _____
   i. Position the patient in high Fowler's. _____
   j. Lubricate the tube. _____

Copyright © 2019, Elsevier Inc. All Rights Reserved.

39. For a patient who is incontinent, how can skin irritation be prevented?

40. What type of ostomy is shown in the graphic?

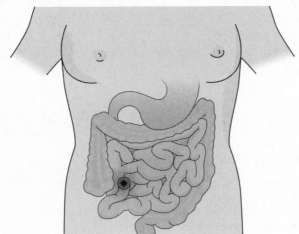

41. The nurse has instilled 30 mL prior to irrigation of the NG tube. The return is 55 mL. How is this fluid recorded?

42. What can you tell the patient about a computed tomography (CT) scan of the abdomen?

43. The patient has had several days of diarrhea and is in danger of becoming dehydrated. What signs would indicate this problem?

Select the best answer for each of the following questions:

44. For a patient with a nasogastric tube who has a painful, distended abdomen, the first most appropriate action by the nurse is to:
    1. remove the tube.
    2. irrigate the tube.
    3. pull the tube out farther.
    4. notify the supervisor.

45. A patient expresses a feeling of mild cramping during the administration of a saline enema. The nurse should first:
    1. discontinue the procedure.
    2. change the solution.
    3. lower the bag to slow the infusion.
    4. allow the solution to cool.

46. The patient begins to cough during the insertion of the nasogastric tube. The nurse should:
    1. remove the tube.
    2. lower the head of the bed.
    3. check the back of the throat.
    4. advance the tube further.

47. A nurse observes a nursing assistant carrying out bowel training with a patient in the extended care facility. The nurse identifies that the assistant requires further instruction when the assistant is:
    1. allowing the patient adequate time in the bathroom.
    2. restricting fluids with breakfast and lunch meals.
    3. pulling the curtain around the patient while on the commode.
    4. taking the patient to the bathroom at regular times throughout the day.

48. For patients who have been prescribed extended bed rest, the prolonged immobility may result in reduced peristalsis and fecal impaction. A nurse is alert to one of the signs of an impaction when the patient experiences:
    1. oozing of liquid stool.
    2. rectal bleeding.
    3. headaches.
    4. increased appetite.

49. A patient has been admitted to an acute care unit with a diagnosis of biliary disease. When assessing the patient's feces, the nurse expects that they will be:
    1. bloody.
    2. pus filled.
    3. black and tarry.
    4. white or clay colored.

50. The nurse is documenting the appearance of the colostomy stoma. The term for a stoma that is above the abdominal skin level is:
    1. budded.
    2. flush.
    3. retracted.
    4. edematous.

51. A nurse is preparing to administer an enema to an adolescent. When assembling the equipment, the nurse will prepare an enema of:
    1. 100–150 mL of fluid.
    2. 200–400 mL of fluid.
    3. 500–700 mL of fluid.
    4. 800–950 mL of fluid.

52. A nurse recognizes that the greatest challenge for skin care will be for a patient with a(n):
    1. ileostomy.
    2. sigmoid colostomy.
    3. descending ostomy.
    4. ileoanal pouch.

Copyright © 2019, Elsevier Inc. All Rights Reserved.

53. A nurse evaluates that a patient has normal bowel sounds by auscultating all four quadrants and finding:
   1. 3 sounds per minute.
   2. 5–35 sounds per minute.
   3. 60 sounds per minute.
   4. no bowel sounds after 1 minute.

54. A nurse instructs a patient who is taking an iron supplement that his stool may be:
   1. red and liquid.
   2. pale and frothy.
   3. mucus filled.
   4. black or tarry.

55. A nurse is caring for a patient with a Salem sump tube for gastric decompression. Which of the following actions by the nurse requires correction?
   1. Clamping off the blue lumen or air vent
   2. Using clean technique to insert the tube
   3. Anchoring the tube to the patient's gown
   4. Keeping the nares lubricated

56. Which of the following is a commonly used antidiarrheal agent?
   1. Loperamide
   2. Bisacodyl
   3. Senna
   4. Colace

57. Further follow up is required if a patient informs the nurse that he regularly uses enemas, but especially if he uses:
   1. Fleet enemas.
   2. tap water enemas.
   3. castile soap enemas.
   4. normal saline enemas.

58. During a digital removal of a fecal impaction, a nurse notes that the patient has bradycardia. The nurse should:
   1. provide oxygen.
   2. discontinue the procedure.
   3. turn the patient on the right side.
   4. instruct the patient to take rapid, deep breaths.

59. In the teaching plan for a patient who will be having a fecal occult blood test, which of the following foods should be noted for producing a false negative result?
   1. Fish
   2. Pasta
   3. Vitamin C
   4. Whole grain bread

60. The laxatives that are considered safest and least irritating are:
   1. emollients.
   2. stimulants.
   3. osmotics.
   4. bulk forming.

STUDY GROUP QUESTIONS

- What is the normal anatomy and physiology of the gastrointestinal system?
- How is bowel elimination influenced by the process of growth and development?
- What are some common bowel elimination problems?
- How are continent and incontinent bowel diversions/ostomies different?
- What is included in the nursing assessment of a patient to determine bowel elimination status?
- What diagnostic tests may be used to determine the presence of bowel elimination disorders?
- How are the critical thinking and nursing processes applied to situations in which patients are experiencing alterations in bowel elimination?
- What nursing interventions may be implemented to promote bowel elimination, comfort, and dignity for patients in the health promotion, acute care, and restorative care settings?
- What information should be included in the teaching plan for patients/families with regard to promotion and/or restoration of bowel elimination?
- What screenings are recommended to determine bowel pathology? When are they recommended to be done?

STUDY CHART

Create concept maps with nursing diagnoses, related assessment data, and nursing interventions for the following: constipation, diarrhea, and incontinence.

Copyright © 2019, Elsevier Inc. All Rights Reserved.

38 Skin Integrity and Wound Care

PRELIMINARY READING

Chapter 38, pp. 1100–1167

CASE STUDIES

1. You are a student nurse assigned to provide care to a patient in an extended care facility. While assisting the patient from the bed to the shower chair, you notice reddened areas on her sacral region, and on both elbows and heels. The skin on these areas is intact, but it is identified as nonblanchable hyperemia.
   a. Identify a nursing diagnosis, patient goal/outcomes, and nursing interventions related to this patient's assessment data.

2. A male patient was involved in an automobile accident which resulted in multiple fractures and the need to have the left arm casted and the left leg placed into traction. In the initial period of hospitalization, the patient also had an indwelling urinary catheter.
   a. Identify the areas that should be assessed for pressure injuries.
   b. Indicate the care that should be provided.

CHAPTER REVIEW

Match the description/definition in Column A with the correct term in Column B.

Column A	Column B
_____ 1. Localized collection of blood under the tissues	a. Induration
_____ 2. Separation of wound layers with protrusion of visceral organs	b. Approximate
_____ 3. Wound edges come together	c. Abrasion
_____ 4. Superficial loss of dermis	d. Laceration
_____ 5. Pressure exerted against the skin when the patient is moved	e. Dehiscence
_____ 6. Hardening of tissue due to edema or inflammation	f. Granulation tissue
_____ 7. Removal of devitalized tissue	g. Hematoma
_____ 8. Torn, jagged damage to dermis and epidermis	h. Evisceration
_____ 9. Separation of skin and tissue layers	i. Debridement
_____ 10. Red, moist tissue consisting of blood vessels and connective tissue	j. Shearing force

Copyright © 2019, Elsevier Inc. All Rights Reserved.

Complete the following:

11. Mark the areas on the body that are common sites for pressure ulcer development.

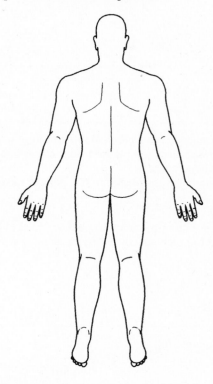

12. Identify the following stages of pressure ulcer development:

a.

Lightly Pigmented   Darkly Pigmented

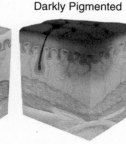

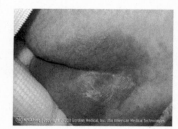

Source: National Pressure Ulcer Advisory Panel (NPUAP), European Pressure Ulcer Advisory Panel (EPUAP) and Pan Pacific Pressure Injury Alliance (PPPIA): *Prevention and treatment of pressure ulcers: quick reference guide*, July 22, 2016.

b.

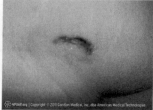

13. Provide an example of an external and an internal contributing factor for pressure ulcer formation.

14. Patients in what age groups are at the highest risk for pressure injuries and sensitivity to heat and cold applications?

15. The major change in an older adult's skin that contributes to pressure ulcer development is:

16. Identify the following related to wound healing.
   a. A clean surgical wound with little tissue loss heals by:

   b. A severe laceration or chronic wound heals by:

17. Identify if the following statements are true or false.
   a. Wounds that are kept moist for several days heal faster than those that are kept dry.

   True _____ False _____

   b. Specimens for wound cultures should be taken from wound areas with clean, healthy skin.

   True _____ False _____

   c. The Centers for Medicare and Medicaid Services (CMS) do not reimburse an acute care facility if a patient with intact skin develops a stage 3–4 pressure injury while hospitalized.

   True _____ False _____

   d. For incontinent patients, underpads and diapers with a plastic outer lining are the best supplies.

   True _____ False _____

   e. The usual wound care in the home environment is performed by the patient or family using sterile technique.

   True _____ False _____

   f. Povidone-iodine (e.g., Betadine), hydrogen peroxide, and acetic acid should not be used to irrigate a clean, granular wound.

   True _____ False _____

   g. High pressure over a short time and low pressure over a long time cause skin breakdown.

   True _____ False _____

Copyright © 2019, Elsevier Inc. All Rights Reserved.

18. Identify a complication of wound healing that is assessed by the nurse in the following examples.
    a. Separation of the layers of the skin with serosanguineous drainage noted
    b. Bluish swelling or mass at the site
    c. Fever, general malaise, and increased white blood cell (WBC) count
    d. Green, odorous local drainage
    e. Decreased blood pressure, increased pulse rate, increased respirations
    f. Visceral organs protruding through abdominal wall
    g. Wound edges swollen, painful, with redness extending from the edges outward

19. a. To ensure that skin inspection is more accurate, the nurse should use:

    b. Identify the methods or indicators that are used for assessing darkly pigmented skin.

20. Identify an example of how each of the following factors influences wound healing.
    a. Age
    b. Obesity
    c. Diabetes
    d. Immunosuppression
    e. Scar tissue
    f. Radiation

21. Match each of the following types of wound drainage with their correct description.

Drainage	Description
a. Serous	1. Pale, more watery, with plasma and red blood cells
b. Sanguineous	2. Thick, yellow, green, or brown with organisms and white blood cells
c. Serosanguineous	3. Clear, watery plasma
d. Purulent	4. Fresh bleeding

22. Provide at least one nursing intervention that should be implemented to prevent pressure injury specifically related to:
    a. Pressure reduction
    b. Skin care

23. Arrange the steps for obtaining a wound culture in correct order.
    a. When tip is saturated, insert into appropriate sterile container. _____
    b. Complete lab slip providing clinical data which includes wound site, time collected and prior antibiotics. _____
    c. Moisten swab with normal saline. _____
    d. While applying pressure, rotate applicator within 1–2 cm^2 of clean wound tissue (try to draw out tissue fluid). _____
    e. Clean wound surface 1 cm^2 with an antiseptic solution. _____

24. A patient with a dirty, penetrating wound is asked by the nurse whether a _____ injection has been received within the last 10 years.

25. Identify how the nurse determines whether a wound is healing.

26. A patient who is sitting out of bed in a chair and requires assistance to move around should be limited to _____ hours sitting and should be repositioned every _____ hour(s).

27. A nurse can reduce friction or shear by:

28. Nursing care of an abrasion or laceration includes:

29. For use of a negative pressure wound therapy system:
    a. The purpose of the therapy is to:
    b. The tube is attached to suction that is usually set at:
    c. The dressing that is used for this system is:
    d. What should be done if the patient verbalizes an increase in discomfort with this treatment?
    e. How often should the system be changed?

Copyright © 2019, Elsevier Inc. All Rights Reserved.

30. For wound irrigation, identify the following that are considered as safe guidelines.
   a. Patient positioning
   b. Syringe size
   c. Angiocath gauge
   d. psi
   e. The syringe should be held how far above the wound?
   f. During an irrigation, the nurse notes sanguineous return. The nurse should:
   g. It is noted that there is retained debris in the wound. The nurse should:
   h. How do you irrigate a deep wound with a very small opening?

31. Identify what is pictured in the following illustrations:

a.

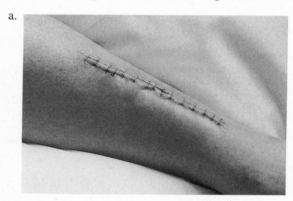

b.

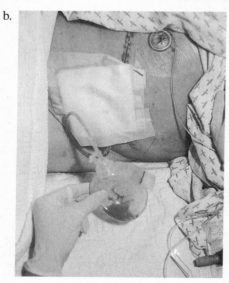

32. Which of the following are correct nursing interventions for elastic bandages? Select all that apply.
   a. Placing the body part to be bandaged in anatomical position _____
   b. Applying a bandage to an extremity from proximal to distal _____
   c. Positioning pins or knots toward the wound _____
   d. Overlapping turns by one-half to two-thirds the width of the bandage _____
   e. Assessing circulation once daily _____

33. Identify the steps in caring for a traumatic wound.

34. Specify whether the following effects are a result of heat (H) therapy, cold (C) therapy or both.
   a. Vasoconstriction _____
   b. Decreased blood viscosity _____
   c. Increased tissue metabolism _____
   d. Decreased muscle tension _____
   e. Increased capillary permeability _____

35. a. Provide an instance in which the application of heat is contraindicated.
   b. Provide an instance in which the application of cold is contraindicated.

36. The usual duration of time for the application of heat or cold is:

37. Which of the following are correct for the application of heat or cold? Select all that apply.
   a. Providing a timer or clock so the patient may help time the application _____
   b. Allowing the patient to adjust the temperature setting _____
   c. Placing the patient in a position that prevents movement away from the temperature source _____
   d. Maintaining the temperature as hot or as cold as the patient is able to stand _____
   e. Applying a heating pad or cold pack directly to the skin _____
   f. Adding hotter solution to a soak to maintain temperature while the patient remains immersed _____

Copyright © 2019, Elsevier Inc. All Rights Reserved.

g. Keeping the rest of the patient draped or covered while receiving treatment _____

38. Using the Braden Scale, what is this patient's risk for pressure injury?

		Score
Sensory	Very limited	_____
Moisture	Occasionally	_____
Activity	Chairfast	_____
Mobility	Very limited	_____
Nutrition	Probably inadequate	_____
Friction/Shear	Potential problem	_____
	Total score	_____
	Patient risk	_____

39. Which of the following are correct for application of a moist dressing? Select all that apply.

a. Wringing out excess moisture from the dressing _____

b. Pouring the solution directly onto the dressing in the wound _____

c. Loosely packing sinus tracks or dead spaces in the wound _____

d. Avoiding the use of secondary dressings _____

e. Using Montgomery ties or straps perpendicular to the wound _____

40. a. Nonblanchable hyperemia is:
b. This assessment signifies:
c. When nonblanchable hyperemia is assessed, the stage is reversible if pressure is relieved.

True _____ False _____

41. Which of the following are correct actions for a postoperative dressing? Select all that apply.

a. Routinely changing the dressing soon after the procedure _____

b. Reinforcing saturated dressings _____

c. Providing the patient with an analgesic 30 minutes before the dressing change _____

d. Expecting inflammation of the wound edges for at least a week after the surgery _____

e. Noting the amount, color, consistency, and odor of wound drainage _____

42. A patient will need to continue to perform dressing changes when he is discharged to his home. Identify the necessary nursing assessments/evaluations before the patient's discharge.

43. Topical skin care for a patient should include: Select all that apply.

a. Massaging reddened areas _____

b. Examining the skin at least daily _____

c. Using a mild cleansing agent _____

d. Keeping the head of the bed at greater than a 30-degree angle _____

e. Applying a moisture barrier product _____

f. Repositioning the patient in the chair every 3 hours _____

44. How are enzyme agents used?

45. Match the following wounds with the type of dressing that is most appropriate.

Wounds	Dressings
a. Maintains moist environment to facilitate wound healing while protecting wound base. _____	1. Gauze
b. Delivers moisture to a wound and is absorptive. _____	2. Transparent film
c. Maintains a moist environment and offers intact skin protection. _____	3. Hydrocolloid

46. The correct way to remove old tape from the skin is to:

47. How can the nurse reduce discomfort during dressing changes?

Copyright © 2019, Elsevier Inc. All Rights Reserved.

48. Identify the correct techniques for the application of a sling. Select all that apply.
   a. Have the patient sit or lie supine for application. _____

   b. Ask the patient to bend the affected arm, bringing the forearm straight across the chest. _____

   c. Position the base of the triangle under the wrist and the point of the triangle at the elbow. _____

   d. Tie the ends at the back of the neck. _____

   e. Make sure that the lower arm is supported at a level above the elbow. _____

49. The desired temperature for a cold soak is _____.

50. For sitz baths:
   a. When are they usually used?
   b. What safety measures are implemented?

51. Name some general safety for prevention and treatment of pressure injuries.

52. The support system of choice for a patient with atelectasis and/or pneumonia is:

53. If there is a chance of splashing during wound care or irrigation, the nurse should use:

Select the best answer for each of the following questions:

54. To avoid pressure injury for an immobilized patient at home, a nurse recommends a surface to use on the bed. A surface type that is low cost and easy to use in the home is a(n):
   1. foam overlay.
   2. water mattress.
   3. air fluidized bed.
   4. low-air-loss surface.

55. For a patient in the extended care facility who has a risk for pressure injuries, a nurse will implement:
   1. massage of reddened skin areas.
   2. movement of the patient in the chair every 3 hours.
   3. maintenance of a position while in bed at 30 degrees or lower.
   4. placement of plastic absorptive pads directly beneath the patient.

56. A patient has experienced a traumatic injury that will require applications of heat. The nurse implements the treatment based on the principle that:
   1. patient response is best to minor temperature adjustments.
   2. the foot and the palm of the hand are the most sensitive to temperature.
   3. long exposures help the patient develop tolerance to the procedure.
   4. patients are more tolerant to temperature changes over a large body surface area.

57. A severely overweight patient has returned to the unit after having major abdominal surgery. When the nurse enters the room, it is evident that the patient has moved or coughed and the wound has eviscerated. The nurse should immediately:
   1. assess vital signs.
   2. contact the physician.
   3. apply light pressure on the exposed organs.
   4. place sterile towels soaked in saline over the area.

58. A patient with a knife protruding from his upper leg is taken into the emergency department. A nurse is waiting for the physician to arrive when a newly hired nurse comes to assist. The nurse delegates the new staff nurse to do all of the following as soon as possible except:
   1. assess vital signs.
   2. remove the knife to cleanse the wound.
   3. wrap a bandage around the knife and injured site.
   4. apply pressure to the surrounding area to stop bleeding.

59. A nurse is assessing a patient's superficial wound and notices that it has very minimal tissue loss and drainage. There are a number of dressings that may be used according to the protocol on the unit. The nurse selects:
   1. gauze.
   2. alginate.
   3. transparent film.
   4. negative pressure wound therapy.

60. A nurse is completing an assessment of the patient's skin integrity and identifies that an area is a full-thickness loss of skin with adipose tissue, slough, and eschar visible. The nurse identifies this stage of pressure injury as:
   1. stage 1.
   2. stage 2.
   3. stage 3.
   4. stage 4.

Copyright © 2019, Elsevier Inc. All Rights Reserved.

61. A patient has a large wound to the sacral area that requires irrigation. The nurse explains to the patient that irrigation will be performed to:
    1. decrease scar formation.
    2. decrease wound drainage.
    3. improve circulation in the wound.
    4. remove debris from the wound.

62. A nurse is working with an older adult patient in an extended care facility. While turning the patient, the nurse notices that there is a reddened area on the patient's coccyx. The nurse implements skin care that includes:
    1. soaking the area with normal saline and baking soda.
    2. using a mild cleansing agent, drying, and applying a protective moisturizer.
    3. washing the area with an astringent and painting it with povidone-iodine solution.
    4. applying a dilute solution of hydrogen peroxide and water and using a heat lamp to dry the area.

63. A patient has a wound to the left lower extremity that has minimal exudates, and granulation tissue and collagen formation. The nurse identifies the healing phase of this wound as:
    1. primary intention.
    2. proliferative phase.
    3. secondary intention.
    4. inflammatory phase.

64. After neurosurgery, a nurse assesses the patient's bandage and finds that there is fresh bleeding coming from the operative site. The nurse describes this drainage to the surgeon as:
    1. serous.
    2. purulent.
    3. sanguineous.
    4. serosanguineous.

65. A patient has a surgical wound on the right upper aspect of the chest that requires cleansing. The nurse implements appropriate aseptic technique by:
    1. opening the cleansing solution with sterile gloves.
    2. moving from the outer region of the wound toward the center.
    3. cleaning the wound twice and discarding the swab.
    4. starting at the drainage site and moving outward with circular motions.

66. A nurse is working in a physician's office and is asked by one of the patients when heat or cold should be applied. In providing an example, the nurse identifies that cold therapy should be applied for the patient with:
    1. a newly fractured ankle.
    2. menstrual cramping.
    3. an infected wound.
    4. degenerative joint disease.

67. A patient will require the application of a binder to provide support to the abdomen. When applying the binder, the nurse uses the principle that the:
    1. binder should be kept loose for patient comfort.
    2. patient should be sitting or standing when it is applied.
    3. patient must maintain adequate ventilatory capacity.
    4. binder replaces the need for underlying bandages or dressings.

68. A nurse is aware that malnutrition places a patient at a greater risk for tissue damage. The patient with the greatest risk is the individual who:
    1. experienced a 7% weight loss in the last month.
    2. is between 45–60 years of age.
    3. has an albumin level of 5 g/100 mL.
    4. has a transferrin level of 120 mg/dL.

69. The agent that is most effective and safest for cleaning a granular wound is:
    1. acetic acid.
    2. normal saline.
    3. povidone-iodine.
    4. hydrogen peroxide.

70. A nurse is working with a patient who has a stage 3, clean pressure injury with significant exudate. The nurse anticipates that which of the following dressings will be used?
    1. Adherent film dressing
    2. Transparent dressing
    3. Calcium alginate dressing
    4. Dry gauze dressing

71. For a patient's optimal nutritional intake that will promote formation of new blood vessels and collagen synthesis, the nurse plans to teach the patient to include a sufficient intake of:
    1. fats.
    2. proteins.
    3. carbohydrates.
    4. fat-soluble vitamins.

72. The nurse notices that the skin surrounding a wound appears macerated. The nurse should:
    1. obtain a wound culture.
    2. monitor lab results.
    3. turn the patient more frequently.
    4. select a different dressing.

Copyright © 2019, Elsevier Inc. All Rights Reserved.

STUDY GROUP QUESTIONS

- What are pressure injuries and what contributes to their development?
- Where are pressure injuries most likely to develop?
- What are the stages of pressure injury development?
- What are the classifications of wounds?
- How do wounds heal?
- What are the possible complications of wound healing?
- How do pressure injuries affect health care costs?
- What tools may be used to predict patients' risks for pressure injuries?
- What should be included in the nursing assessment of patients to determine their risk for pressure injuries?
- How are wounds managed in both emergency and nonemergency health care settings?
- What types of drainage may be seen in wounds?
- How are wound cultures obtained?
- How can the nurse prevent pressure ulcer development?

- What nursing interventions may be implemented to treat pressure injuries and wounds?
- What are the procedures for dressing changes and wound care?
- What criteria are used in the selection of dressings and sutures or staples?
- What are the principles involved in heat and cold therapy, including patient safety?
- What information should be included in patient/family teaching for prevention and treatment of pressure injuries, wound care, and use of heat and cold therapy?

STUDY ACTIVITY

When on a medical unit, find the supplies that are used for wound care, including different types of dressings and cleansing agents, in order to become familiar with the products.

Copyright © 2019, Elsevier Inc. All Rights Reserved.

39 Sensory Alterations

Copyright © 2019, Elsevier Inc. All Rights Reserved.

PRELIMINARY READING

Chapter 39, pp. 1168–1186

CASE STUDIES

1. You are making a home visit to a patient with diabetes mellitus who is losing his eyesight (diabetic retinopathy).
   a. What interventions may be implemented with the patient to assist in maintaining adequate sensory stimulation?
   b. How can you promote a safe environment for him?

2. You have been assigned to care for a patient in the intensive care unit (ICU).
   a. What sensory alterations may this patient experience?
   b. How can you prevent the occurrence of these alterations or reduce their impact?

3. The older adult patient seems to be repeating questions and parts of the conversation. She also seems to be answering inappropriately to questions, smiling and nodding her head in approval. The patient is still able to perform ADLs, but there appears to be a sensory issue.
   a. What issue do you suspect?
   b. How can you assist this patient to improve her sensory status?

CHAPTER REVIEW

Complete the following:

1. Identify other terms for the following:
   a. Sight
   b. Hearing
   c. Taste
   d. Smell
   e. Touch
   f. Position sense

2. Identify one of the major diseases that can lead to visual impairment.

3. Identify at least one factor that can lead to each of the following *Disturbed Sensory Perception* diagnoses, and indicate possible patient responses, signs, and symptoms:
   a. Sensory deprivation
   b. Sensory overload

4. Provide the correct term for each of the following:
   a. A buildup of ear wax in the external auditory canal
   b. Hearing loss associated with aging
   c. Opacity of the lens resulting in blurred vision
   d. Decreased salivary production or dry mouth

5. Identify how the following factors may influence sensory function:
   a. Age: older adulthood
   b. Medications
   c. Smoking
   d. Environment

6. How can a nurse evaluate a patient's vision and hearing during routine interactions or care?

7. For visual and hearing impairments in children:
   a. A common cause of blindness is:
   b. What information should be included when teaching parents about eyesight safety?
   c. Common causes of hearing impairment in children:

8. Orientation to the environment for a patient with a sensory deficit should include:

9. Identify a way that a nurse can modify sensory stimulation in the health care environment.

Copyright © 2019, Elsevier Inc. All Rights Reserved.

10. A nurse may communicate with a hearing-impaired patient by:

11. For a patient with cataracts, the nurse anticipates which of the following signs and symptoms? Select all that apply.

    a. Cloudy vision _____

    b. Eye pain _____

    c. Glare _____

    d. Burning sensation _____

    e. Poor night vision _____

    f. Double vision _____

12. Indicate how a nurse may assist patients with the following deficits to adapt their home environments for safety:
    a. Hearing deficit
    b. Diminished sense of smell
    c. Diminished sense of touch

13. Identify a goal/outcome for a patient with a nursing diagnosis of *Disturbed Sensory Perception*.

14. In relation to screening for sensory deficits:
    a. Provide an example of a general screening that is conducted to determine visual and/or auditory deficits.
    b. The recommendation of frequency for hearing screenings is:

15. Which of the following are appropriate in promoting sensory stimulation in the home environment? Select all that apply.
    a. Reducing glare by using sheer curtains on windows _____

    b. Using pale colors on surfaces _____

    c. Serving bland foods with similar textures _____

    d. Using a pocket magnifier _____

    e. Introducing fragrant flowers _____

    f. Playing recorded music with high-frequency sound _____

16. A patient has gone to the local walk-in emergency center with flu-like symptoms. After seeing the physician, the patient shows the nurse the prescriptions the physician has written. The patient should be informed that ototoxicity may occur with the administration of which of the following medications? Select all that apply.

    a. Furosemide _____

    b. Vitamin C _____

    c. Acetaminophen _____

    d. Vancomycin _____

    e. Cough suppressant with codeine _____

    f. Aspirin _____

17. Identify at least one rationale for why a patient may not use his or her hearing aid.

18. A patient with a diminished tactile sense may be assisted with hygiene and grooming by:

19. What are the signs and symptoms associated with Ménierè's disease?

20. The nurse is caring for a patient with a hearing aid. What is included in the care for this patient and the assistive device?

21. Behaviors that are specific for an adult with a visual impairment include (select all that apply):

    a. Poor coordination _____

    b. Rocking _____

    c. Squinting _____

    d. No reaction to being touched _____

    e. Accidental falls _____

    f. Increase in appetite _____

22. Identify community resources where a patient with a sensory impairment may be referred.

Copyright © 2019, Elsevier Inc. All Rights Reserved.

23. The occupational health nurse wants to promote safety for the employees. What general safety measures may be implemented by the nurse in a work environment?

24. Provide an example of a patient who may experience sensory deprivation.

25. In assisting the visually impaired patient to ambulate, the nurse should (select all that apply):
    a. warn the patient when approaching doorways. _____

    b. stand on the nondominant/injured side _____
    c. position the patient so that they are directly behind you. _____
    d. walk one-half step ahead and slightly to the side. _____

    e. have the patient grasp your waist. _____
    f. walk at a comfortable pace. _____
    g. use a gait belt for unstable patients. _____

26. Which individuals are at the highest risk for occupational hearing loss?

27. How can sensory loss affect an individual's life?

Select the best answer for each of the following questions:

28. An expected outcome for a patient with an auditory deficit should include:
    1. minimizing use of affected sense(s).
    2. preventing additional sensory losses.
    3. promoting the patient's acceptance of dependency.
    4. controlling the environment to reduce sensory stimuli.

29. A nurse is working with patients at the senior day care center and recognizes that changes in sensory status may influence the older adult's eating patterns. For patients who are experiencing changes in their dietary intake, the nurse will assess for:
    1. presbycusis.
    2. xerostomia.
    3. vestibular ataxia.
    4. peripheral neuropathy.

30. Parents arrive at the pediatric clinic with their 1 ½-year-old child. The parents ask the nurse if there are signs that may indicate that the child is not able to hear well. The nurse explains to the parents that they should be alert to the child:
    1. awakening to loud noises.
    2. responding reflexively to sounds.
    3. having delayed speech development.
    4. remaining calm when unfamiliar people approach.

31. A nurse is assessing a patient for a potential gustatory impairment. This may be indicated if the patient has a(n):
    1. weight loss.
    2. blank look or stare.
    3. increased sensitivity to odors.
    4. period of excessive clumsiness or dizziness.

32. Which of the following is a priority safety measure in the acute care environment for a patient with a sensory deficit?
    1. Encouraging the family to visit the patient
    2. Referring the patient to a support group
    3. Determining the patient's medical history
    4. Orienting the patient to the surroundings

33. A responsive patient had eye surgery, and patches have been temporarily placed on both eyes for protection. The evening meal has arrived, and the nurse will be assisting the patient. In this circumstance, the nurse should:
    1. feed the patient the entire meal.
    2. encourage family members to feed the patient.
    3. allow the patient to be totally independent and feed himself.
    4. orient the patient to the locations of the foods on the plate and provide the utensils.

34. After a cerebrovascular accident (CVA or stroke), a patient is found to have receptive aphasia. The nurse may assist this patient with communication by:
    1. obtaining a referral for a speech therapist.
    2. using a system of simple gestures and repeated behaviors.
    3. providing the patient with a letter chart to use to answer questions.
    4. offering the patient a notepad and pen to write down questions and concerns.

35. A patient has been diagnosed with glaucoma. The nurse anticipates that the patient will report a history of:
    1. severe redness and itching of the eyes.
    2. cloudy and blurred vision.
    3. painless loss of peripheral vision.
    4. dark spaces blocking forward vision and distortion of lines.

Copyright © 2019, Elsevier Inc. All Rights Reserved.

36. A mother is taking her newborn for his first physical examination. She expresses concern because during her pregnancy she may have been exposed to an infectious disease, and the baby's hearing could be affected. The nurse inquires if the patient was exposed to:
    1. rubella.
    2. pneumonia.
    3. tuberculosis.
    4. a urinary tract infection.

37. For a patient with a hearing deficit, the best way for the nurse to communicate is to:
    1. approach the patient from the side.
    2. use visible facial expressions.
    3. shout or speak very loudly to the patient.
    4. repeat the entire conversation if it is not totally understood.

38. The school nurse recognizes that the most common type of visual disorder in children is:
    1. glaucoma.
    2. retinal detachment.
    3. nearsightedness.
    4. macular degeneration.

39. Because of the possibility of diminished independence for the patient with sensory losses, an important and specific ethical standard for the nurse to follow is the preservation of:
    1. autonomy.
    2. fidelity.
    3. justice.
    4. nonmaleficence.

40. Which of the following needs to be corrected in the room for the patient with a visual impairment?
    1. The call light is left on the bedside stand.
    2. The patient's tissues are on the patient's lap.
    3. The path to the bathroom is cleared of equipment.
    4. The patient's slippers are on the floor where the patient left them when returning to bed.

STUDY GROUP QUESTIONS

- What are the human senses and their functions?
- What factors influence sensory function?
- What are some common sensory alterations?
- What types of patients are at risk for developing sensory alterations?
- How should a nurse assess a patient's sensory function?
- What behaviors or changes in lifestyle patterns or socialization may indicate a sensory alteration?
- How can a nurse promote sensory function and prevent injury and isolation in the health promotion and acute and restorative care settings?
- What screening processes are used to determine the presence of sensory alterations?
- How may the family/significant others be involved in the care of a patient with a sensory alteration?
- What information should be included in patient/family teaching for promotion of sensory function and prevention of injury?

Copyright © 2019, Elsevier Inc. All Rights Reserved.

40 Surgical Patient

PRELIMINARY READING

Chapter 40, pp. 1187–1237

CASE STUDIES

1. Your patient is scheduled to have extensive abdominal surgery with a large, midline incision.
   a. How can you assist this patient to promote respiratory function postoperatively?

2. A patient is having outpatient surgery.
   a. How may preoperative teaching be conducted, and what information should be included?
   b. The patient does not appear to have an understanding of the surgery or possible complications. What should you do?

3. While completing the preoperative checklist, you discover that a patient's temperature is 101°F.
   a. What action should be taken?

4. A patient insists that his good luck medallion must go with him everywhere, even to surgery.
   a. What should you do?
   b. What personal items or prosthetics should be accounted for prior to surgery?

5. A patient had laparoscopic surgery on his right knee and is going to be discharged to his home. His wife and young children have visited often during his hospital stay.
   a. What general information do you need in order to prepare the patient and the family for the discharge?

6. The patient has come into the ambulatory surgery center in the hospital for hernia repair. Upon admission to the PACU, the patient's oxygen saturation is 88% and he is not easy to arouse. There is no evidence of bleeding on the lower right abdominal dressing and no distention.
   a. What should you do for this patient in the PACU?
   b. After 3 hours, the patient has still not had any urinary output. What options are available?

CHAPTER REVIEW

Match the description/definition in Column A with the correct term in Column B.

	Column A	Column B
_____	1. Performed on the basis of the patient's choice; not essential for health	a. Palliative surgery
_____	2. Involves extensive reconstruction or alteration in body parts; poses risks to well-being	b. Transplant surgery
_____	3. Relieves or reduces intensity of disease symptoms; will not produce cure	c. Major surgery
_____	4. Must be done immediately to save life or preserve function of body part	d. Ablative surgery
_____	5. Surgical exploration that allows physician to confirm medical status; may involve removal of body tissue for analysis	e. Cosmetic surgery
_____	6. Performed to improve personal appearance	f. Emergency surgery
_____	7. Amputation or removal of diseased body part	g. Elective surgery
_____	8. Performed to replace malfunctioning organs or structures	h. Diagnostic surgery

Copyright © 2019, Elsevier Inc. All Rights Reserved.

Complete the following:

9. a. In relation to the operative experience, a patient who smokes cigarettes is at a greater risk for:

b. Postoperative care for this patient will require more aggressive:

10. a. Identify a medical condition that may increase a patient's surgical risk.

b. Malignant hyperthermia is:

c. The pregnant patient is at greater risk because of:

11. Identify an example of how changes in each of the following body systems place the older adult patient at risk during surgery.
a. Cardiovascular
b. Pulmonary
c. Renal
d. Neurological

12. Obesity places a patient at greater risk for surgery as a result of:

13. Identify a consideration for surgical patients who are taking the following medications.
a. Insulin
b. Antibiotics
c. NSAIDs
d. Corticosteroids

14. a. Provide two examples of information that is usually included in preoperative teaching.
b. What is involved in prehabilitation?

15. Identify a routine screening test that may be ordered for a patient.

16. Identify the commonly used types of preoperative medications.

17. Identify two nursing diagnoses and related goals that may be formulated for a patient who will be having his or her first surgery.

18. The patient is going to receive general anesthesia for the surgical procedure. Specify the general NPO criteria for the following.

a. No food or fluids _____ hours before surgery

b. No meat or fried foods _____ hours before surgery

c. The patient accidentally ingests some food within the NPO restricted time frame. What do you do?

19. Identify the adverse effects associated with the following types of anesthesia.
a. General anesthesia
b. Regional anesthesia
c. Local anesthesia
d. Moderate (conscious) sedation

20. Which of the following preoperative interventions are appropriate? Select all that apply.
a. Completing bowel preparation before GI surgery

_____

b. Shaving the surgical site with a razor _____

c. Providing antimicrobial soap for bathing _____

d. Removing the patient's wig _____

e. Leaving artificial fingernails intact _____

f. Removing a hearing aid when the patient gets to the operating room (OR) _____

21. In the presurgical care unit (PSCU) and OR, how is verification done to determine:
a. Right patient
b. Right body part
c. Right frame of mind of the patient
d. Preparation for surgery

22. Identify whether the following tasks are responsibilities of the circulating nurse (C) or scrub nurse (S).
a. Completion of preoperative assessments/verification

_____

b. Application of sterile drapes _____

c. Establishment of the intraoperative plan of care

_____

d. Calculation of blood loss and urinary output

_____

e. Provision of sterile equipment for the surgeon

_____

f. Documentation of the procedure _____

g. Maintenance of the sterile field _____

23. For the following, identify a nursing intervention for intraoperative patient care.
a. Prevention of injury
b. Maintenance of patient's body temperature
c. Prevention of infection

24. Identify a specific nursing intervention to prevent the following postoperative complications.
a. Pulmonary stasis
b. Venous stasis
c. Wound infection
d. Gastrointestinal stasis

Copyright © 2019, Elsevier Inc. All Rights Reserved.

25. Which of the following assessment findings for a patient in the postanesthesia care unit (PACU) signify that the adult patient is qualified to be discharged from the unit? Select all that apply.

a. Oxygen saturation 96% _____

b. Rales on auscultation _____

c. Pulse rate 110 beats per minute _____

d. Bilateral peripheral pulses _____

e. Abdominal distention _____

f. Response to verbal stimuli _____

g. Sluggish hand grasp and pupillary response _____

h. Quarter-size sanguineous spot maintained on incisional dressing _____

i. 30 mL per hour urinary output _____

26. A nurse is aware that a patient should void within _____ hours after surgery. For the patient who has not voided, what should the nurse do?

27. a. After general anesthesia, postoperative oral intake usually begins with an order for a _____ (diet).

b. This diet is usually followed by a _____ (diet), then a _____.

28. With regard to postoperative wound healing and care, which of the following statements are correct? Select all that apply.

a. The surgical dressing is changed after the patient leaves the PACU. _____

b. Any visible drainage on the surgical dressing should be marked. _____

c. The patient who has an order for an oral analgesic should be medicated 30 minutes before an uncomfortable dressing change. _____

d. Redness, warmth, and edema should be expected at the incision site. _____

e. Wound drainage should be measured once a day. _____

f. The patient should be draped during a dressing change to minimize exposure. _____

29. a. The patient in the illustration is demonstrating the use of a(n):

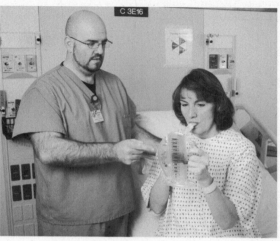

b. This device is used to prevent:

30. For a patient who will be alert during a surgical procedure, what support should be provided by the nurse?

31. Identify examples of routine postoperative patient assessments and interventions.

32. What physical signs and symptoms are indicative of a latex allergy?

33. The American Society of Anesthesiologists recommends that postoperative analgesics be administered:

34. Indicate which of the following are appropriate interventions in the postanesthesia care unit (PACU). Select all that apply.

a. Irrigating an existing N/G tube with normal saline. _____

b. Providing oral fluids. _____

c. Measuring I&O. _____

d. Yelling loudly to arouse the patient. _____

e. Checking for bleeding at the surgical site. _____

f. Administering analgesics. _____

185

Copyright © 2019, Elsevier Inc. All Rights Reserved.

35. Research indicates that the use of preventive measures will decrease the incidence of postoperative wound infection. Identify at least three of those interventions.

36. Which of the following interventions are appropriate for the older adult in the postoperative phase?
    a. Verify an order for subcutaneous heparin if the patient is on bedrest for more than 24 hours. _____
    b. Place the patient in a bed or room that is closer to the nurses' station. _____
    c. Use teaching materials with large print. _____
    d. Determine the need for a stool softener and/or extra fiber. _____
    e. Double the normal intake of iron. _____
    f. Provide pain medication after uncomfortable procedures. _____

37. For the use of an incentive spirometer, place the steps in the correct order.
    a. After a maximum inspiration, patient should hold breath for 2–3 seconds and exhale slowly. _____
    b. Set marker on spirometer at the maximum inspiration point achieved by patient to establish postoperative target. _____
    c. Position patient in sitting position in chair or in reclining position with head of bed elevated at least 45 degrees. _____
    d. Instruct patient to breathe normally for a short period and repeat process 10 times every hour while awake. _____
    e. Instruct patient to exhale completely and place mouthpiece so that lips completely cover it and inhale slowly, maintaining constant flow through unit. _____

38. How can the nurse maintain a patient's self-image during the perioperative experience?

39. To promote wound healing, the patient should have at least _____ kcal/day, along with additional:

40. What information is collected during a preoperative nursing history?

41. a. Patients may take oral medications with sips of water preoperatively if ordered by the health care provider.

    True _____ False _____

    b. Current evidence indicates that bowel preparation is no longer needed for most patients and procedures.

    True _____ False _____

    c. A patient cannot refuse surgery or treatment after giving written consent.

    True _____ False _____

    d. The patient can sign the informed consent after receiving preoperative sedatives.

    True _____ False _____

42. What is the purpose of the "time out" prior to starting the surgical procedure?

43. One of the complications after abdominal surgery can be a loss of function of the intestine.
    a. What is this called?
    b. How can you determine if the patient is having this problem?

44. Which of the following are appropriate measures in the postoperative period? Select all that apply.
    a. Place the patient's arms across the chest. _____
    b. Suction to elicit the gag reflex. _____
    c. Encourage diaphragmatic breathing. _____
    d. Keep patients in bed as long as possible. _____
    e. Maintain pain control. _____

45. The patient has been admitted to the PACU following surgery. You are assessing to see if there are signs of hemorrhage. Where should you check?

46. If a painful stimulus is needed to arouse the patient in the PACU, the nurse should:

Copyright © 2019, Elsevier Inc. All Rights Reserved.

47. Pain management is a priority in the postoperative phase.
    a. When do patients tend to experience the most pain after surgery?
    b. What patient signs, symptoms, or behaviors may indicate that the patient is in pain?
    c. What are the recommendations for postoperative analgesia?
    d. What are some side effects of pain medication?

48. What measures should be taken to prevent deep vein thrombosis after surgery?

49. You are preparing the patient's room on the surgical unit for his return from the PACU. What equipment/supplies will you need?

50. The patient has been admitted to the PACU after surgery.
    a. What should be included in the handoff communication from the OR nurse?
    b. What monitoring should be done for the patient while in the PACU?

Select the best answer for each of the following questions:

51. A nurse is starting the preparations for a patient who is having surgery tomorrow morning. The nurse prepares to have the consent form completed. The nurse recognizes that informed consent:
    1. is valid if the patient is disoriented.
    2. is signed by the patient after the administration of preoperative medications.
    3. indicates that the patient is aware of the procedure and its possible complications.
    4. requires that the nurse provide information about the surgery before the consent can be signed.

52. A patient is taken to PACU after surgery. A nurse is assessing the patient and is alert to the indication of a postoperative hemorrhage if the patient exhibits:
    1. restlessness.
    2. warm, dry skin.
    3. a slow, steady pulse rate.
    4. a decreased respiratory rate.

53. The nurse is checking the urinary output of a young child who weighs 50 pounds. Based on this measurement, the expected hourly urinary output should be
    1. 5–10 mL.
    2. 12–20 mL.
    3. 23–46 mL.
    4. 50–70 mL.

54. A nurse is completing the preoperative checklist for a woman who will be having surgery. The nurse determines that the surgeon and anesthesiologist should be informed of which of the patient's laboratory results?
    1. Hemoglobin level: 10 g/dL
    2. Potassium level: 4.2 mEq/L
    3. Platelet count: 210,000/mm^3
    4. Prothrombin time: 11 seconds

55. A patient has received a spinal anesthetic during the surgical procedure. The nurse is alert to possible complications of the anesthetic and is assessing the patient for a:
    1. rash.
    2. headache.
    3. nephrotoxic response.
    4. hyperthermic response.

56. An adult patient is being evaluated for transfer from the PACU to the patient's unit. The nurse determines that the patient will be approved for transfer if the patient exhibits:
    1. increased wound drainage.
    2. pulse oximetry of 95%.
    3. respirations of 36 breaths per minute.
    4. nonpalpable peripheral pulses.

57. A patient is scheduled to have abdominal surgery later in the morning. At 9:00 a.m., while completing the preoperative checklist, the nurse recognizes the need to contact the surgeon immediately. The nurse has identified that the patient:
    1. received an enema at 6:00 a.m.
    2. admitted to recent substance abuse.
    3. ate a hamburger two evenings ago at 6:00 p.m.
    4. has bowel sounds in all four quadrants of the abdomen.

58. A patient is being positioned in the PACU after surgery. Unless contraindicated, the nurse should place the patient:
    1. prone.
    2. in high Fowler's.
    3. supine with arms across the chest.
    4. on the side with the face turned downward.

59. When a patient first arrives at PACU, the nurse will:
    1. provide oral fluids.
    2. allow the patient to sleep.
    3. provide a warm blanket.
    4. remove the urinary catheter.

Copyright © 2019, Elsevier Inc. All Rights Reserved.

60. A nurse is visiting a patient who had surgery 9 hours ago. The nurse asks if the patient has voided, and the patient responds negatively. The bladder scan shows retained urine and the bladder is palpable. At this time, the nurse:
    1. provides more oral fluids.
    2. inserts an IV and administers fluids.
    3. obtains an order for straight catheterization.
    4. recognizes that this is a normal outcome.

61. During a patient assessment in the PACU, a nurse finds that the patient's operative site is swollen and appears tight. The nurse suspects:
    1. infection.
    2. hemorrhage.
    3. lymphedema.
    4. subcutaneous emphysema.

62. An immediate postoperative priority in providing nursing care for a patient is:
    1. airway patency.
    2. relief of pain.
    3. sufficient circulation to the extremities.
    4. prevention of wound infection.

63. A 54-year-old patient is scheduled to have a gastric resection. The nurse informs the surgeon preoperatively of the patient's history of:
    1. a tonsillectomy at age 10.
    2. employment as a telephone repair person.
    3. smoking two packs of cigarettes per day.
    4. taking acetaminophen for minor body aches.

64. A patient has been taking an anticoagulant at home. The patient is going to be admitted for a surgical procedure, and the nurse anticipates that this prescribed medication will be:
    1. administered as usual.
    2. increased in dose immediately before the procedure.
    3. reduced in dose by half immediately before the procedure.
    4. discontinued at least 2 days before the procedure.

65. During the intraoperative phase, a nurse's responsibility is reflected in the statement:
    1. "I think that the patient requires more information about the procedure and its consequences."
    2. "There seems to be a missing sponge, so a recount must be done to see that all of the sponges were removed."
    3. "The patient has signed the request. I will prepare the medications and then get the record completed."
    4. "The patient appears reactive and stable. Dressing to wound is dry and intact. Analgesic administered per order."

66. A nurse is assisting a patient with postoperative exercises. The patient tells the nurse, "Blowing into this thing [incentive spirometer] is a waste of time." The nurse explains to the patient that the specific purpose of this therapy is to:
    1. stimulate the cough reflex.
    2. promote lung expansion.
    3. increase pulmonary circulation.
    4. directly remove excess secretions from the respiratory tract.

67. A patient is scheduled for surgery, and a nurse is completing the final areas of the preoperative checklist. After administering the preoperative medications, the nurse should:
    1. assist the patient to void.
    2. obtain the informed consent.
    3. prepare the skin at the surgical site.
    4. place the side rails up on the bed or stretcher.

68. At the ambulatory surgery center, a patient is having surgery using general anesthesia. The nurse will expect this patient to:
    1. ambulate immediately after being admitted to the recovery area.
    2. meet all of the identified criteria in order to be discharged home.
    3. remain in the phase I recovery area longer than a hospitalized patient.
    4. receive large amounts of oral fluids immediately upon entering the recovery area.

69. A nurse is preparing a patient for surgery and recognizes that the greatest risk of bleeding is for the patient with:
    1. diabetes mellitus.
    2. emphysema.
    3. thrombocytopenia.
    4. immunodeficiency syndrome.

70. A patient has a nasogastric tube in place after surgery and complains to the nurse of nausea. The nurse should first:
    1. remove the NG tube.
    2. provide oral fluids.
    3. move the patient side to side.
    4. irrigate the tube with normal saline.

71. Which of the following individuals is most at risk for postoperative wound infection?
    1. A pregnant patient
    2. A patient who smokes cigarettes
    3. A patient with poorly controlled diabetes
    4. A patient experiencing periods of sleep apnea

Copyright © 2019, Elsevier Inc. All Rights Reserved.

72. A patient's surgeon has previously discussed the procedure with the patient, but she has a few more questions. The best way for the nurse to approach this is to first:
    1. refer the patient back to the surgeon.
    2. determine what the patient has been told already.
    3. provide details of what the procedure will be like.
    4. get the consent form for the patient to read.

73. The nurse is alert for signs of a postoperative wound infection:
    1. within 24 hours of the surgery.
    2. 1–2 days after the surgery.
    3. 3–6 days after the surgery.
    4. 2 weeks following the surgery.

74. Following surgery, the patient is suspected of having a pulmonary embolism. This is determined by the patient experiencing:
    1. restlessness, chills.
    2. dyspnea, sudden chest pain.
    3. hypotension, nausea.
    4. productive cough, crackles in the lungs.

75. Which of the following are associated with postoperative delirium?
    1. Demonstrating quick-changing emotions and irritability
    2. Having organized thinking and speech
    3. Being awake during the day and sleeping at night
    4. Being continent of urine and stool

STUDY GROUP QUESTIONS

- How are surgeries classified?
- What are some surgical risk factors, and why do they increase the patient's risk?
- How does the incision site influence a patient's recovery?
- How may previous surgical experiences influence the patient's expectations of surgery?

- What general information should be included in preoperative teaching?
- What is the purpose of the preoperative exercises that are explained and demonstrated to patients?
- What preoperative assessments should be made by a nurse?
- What are some common preoperative diagnostic tests that may be ordered for a patient?
- What is prehabilitation and what are the benefits to the patient?
- What nursing interventions are implemented in the preoperative care of patients?
- How does a nurse prepare and assist a patient in the acute care setting on the day of surgery?
- What are the roles of nurses in the operating room and in the recovery setting?
- What interventions are implemented to maintain patient safety and well-being in the operating room and postanesthesia care area?
- What nursing care is critical in the immediate postoperative stage?
- How can the nurse determine the presence of postoperative complications? What nursing interventions should be implemented to prevent these complications?
- What are the similarities and differences between preanesthesia and postanesthesia care for patients in the acute care and ambulatory surgery settings?
- What general information should be included in postoperative teaching for patients/families in the acute care and ambulatory surgery settings?
- How may the family/significant other be involved in the patient's perioperative experience?

STUDY CHART

Create a study chart on *Surgical Risk Factors* that identifies how age, obstructive sleep apnea (OSA), nutritional status, obesity, immunocompetence, fluid/electrolyte balance, radiation treatments, adrenocortical stress, depression, and pregnancy may affect the patient's perioperative experience.

189

Copyright © 2019, Elsevier Inc. All Rights Reserved.

ELSEVIER elsevier.com

Recommended
Shelving Classification
**Nursing Fundamentals
and Skills**

ISBN 978-0-323-53303-4

9 780323 533034